Handbook of psychiatric nursing for primary care

Handbook of psychiatric nursing for primary care

CW Allwood
CA Gagiano
AC Gmeiner
S van Wyk

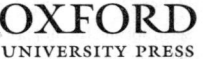

OXFORD

UNIVERSITY PRESS

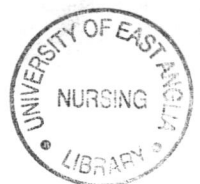

OXFORD
UNIVERSITY PRESS

Great Clarendon Street, Oxford OX2 6DP

Oxford University Press is a department of the University of Oxford.
It furthers the University's objective of excellence in research, scholarship,
and education by publishing worldwide in

Oxford New York

Auckland Bangkok Buenos Aires Cape Town Chennai
Dar es Salaam Delhi Hong Kong Istanbul Karachi Kolkata
Kuala Lumpur Madrid Melbourne Mexico City Mumbai Nairobi
São Paulo Shanghai Singapore Taipei Tokyo Toronto

and an associated company in Berlin

Oxford is a registered trade mark of Oxford University Press
in the UK and certain other countries

Published in South Africa
by Oxford University Press Southern Africa, Cape Town

Handbook of psychiatric nursing for primary care

ISBN 0 19 578050 7

Commissioning editor: Arthur Attwell
Editor: Emily Bowles
Designer: Mark Standley
Medical proofreader: Claire Irving

Published by Oxford University Press Southern Africa
PO Box 12119, N1 City, 7463, Cape Town, Southern Africa

Set in 9pt on 11pt Utopia by RHT desktop publishing, Durbanville
Reproduction by RHT desktop publishing, Durbanville
Cover reproduction by The Image Bureau
Printed and bound by ABC Press

02332572

Contents

List of contributors

Contributors

CW Allwood   MD Psychiatry
                      Associate Professor and Acting Head of the Department
                      of Psychiatry, University of theWitwatersrand

CA Gagiano   MD Psychiatry
                      Professor and Head of the Department of Psychiatry,
                      University of the Orange Free State

AC Gmeiner   M. Cur, PhD Psychiatric Nursing
                      Associate Professor, Department of Nursing Science,
                      Rand Afrikaans University

S van Wyk   M. Cur, PhD Psychiatric Nursing
                      Contract Lecturer, Rand Afrikaans University

This book is adapted from and builds on the *Handbook of Psychiatry for Primary Care*, edited by Allwood and Gagiano, and to which the following people were contributors. The editors and publisher are grateful to them for their contribution, in this adapted edition, to the *Handbook of psychiatric nursing for primary care*.

AJ Bentley   BSc, MB BCh
                      SleepWake Laboratories

M Berk   MB BCh, MMed Psychiatry, FC Psychiatry,
                      PhD, Associate Professor, Department of Psychiatry,
                      University of the Witwatersrand

W Bodemer   MMed Psychiatry, MD
                      Professor and Head of the Department of Psychiatry,
                      University of Pretoria

C Bouwer   MB ChB, BA, MSc, MRCP, MMed Psychiatry, Senior
                      Lecturer, Department of Psychological Medicine,
                      University of Otago, New Zealand

FJW Calitz   DPhil
                      Principal Clinical Psychologist, Department of
                      Psychiatry, University of the Orange Free State

J Chabalala   FC Psychiatry
                      Head of Psychiatric Services, Northern Province

H Faul   FC Psychiatry (SA)
                      Psychiatrist in private practice

VU Fritz
MB Ch, FCP (SA), PhD (Med), FRCP (London)
Professor and Head of the Department of Neurology, Johannesburg Hospital

DH Gould
MA Social Science, Senior Clinical Psychologist, Community Mental Health Services

GAD Hart
MD Psychiatry
Emeritus Professor, Department of Psychiatry, University of the Witwatersrand

J Hull
MA Psychology
Clinical Psychologist in private practice

L Koopowitz
FC Psychiatry
Consultant Psychiatrist, Adelaide, Australia

AJ Lasich
MB ChB, DPM, FC Psychiatry (SA)
Associate Professor and Acting Head, Department of Psychiatry, University of Natal

JF le Roux
MA Psychology
Senior Clincial Psychologist and Lecturer, Department of Psychiatry, University of the Orange Free State

DL Mkize
MMed Psychiatry
Professor and Head of the Department of Psychiatry and Human Behavioural Sciences, Unitra

CD Molteno
PhD
Professor of Mental Handicap, Department of Psychiatry, University of Cape Town

MG Nair
MB ChB, MMed Psychiatry, FC Psychiatry (SA), MD Psychiatry, Deputy Head, Department of Psychiatry, University of Natal

AJ O'Neill-Kerr
FC Psychiatry (SA)
Consultant Psychiatrist, Princess Marina Hospital, Northampton, UK

WP Pienaar
MD Psychiatry
Senior Lecturer, Department of Psychiatry, University of Stellenbosch

FCV Potocnick
MB ChB, MMed Psychiatry, Dip. Mid. (COG), FC Psychiatry (SA), Senior Lecturer, Department of Psychiatry, University of Stellenbosch

HW Pretorius	MMed Psychiatry, MD Associate Professor, Department of Psychiatry, University of Pretoria
TE Rangaka	MMed Psychiatry Community Psychiatrist, Gauteng
JL Roos	MMed Psychiatry, MD Associate Professor, Department of Psychiatry, University of Pretoria
SD Saffer	FRCP (London) Professor and Head of the Department of Neurology, Baragwanath Hospital
SL Seape	FC Psychiatry (SA) Consultant Psychiatrist, Baragwanath Hospital
DJ Stein	BSc, MB ChB, FRCPC, Director of Research, Department of Psychiatry, University of Stellenbosch
PHJJ van Rensburg	MD Psychiatry Professor, Department of Psychiatry, University of the Orange Free State
T Zabow	FC Psychiatry Associate Professor and Deputy Head, Department of Psychiatry, University of Cape Town

PART I
Introduction to mental illness

1 Primary mental health care in South Africa

World literature, as well as local experience, shows that a considerable number of people present to primary health care (PHC) clinics with significant mental health problems, most commonly anxiety and depressive disorders. The literature also shows that there is considerable under-detection of these conditions at PHC level (Clews and Thom, 1999). They cause significant suffering and disability, and some real risk of mortality. Most of these conditions are highly treatable. Staff working in PHC clinics can be trained to identify, manage, and appropriately refer patients with such problems.

At the same time, in South Africa, mental health services have been vertical and separate from other health services. These services have concentrated on dealing with patients with severe mental illness, such as schizophrenia, bipolar mood disorder, and dementia. They have been mainly hospital- and institution-based, and custodial. However, severe mental illnesses, although they tend to be chronic and require long-term treatment, account for less than 10 per cent of the total burden of mental illness. Where community services have been developed, they have mainly concentrated on providing maintenance medication to patients with severe mental illness, who have been discharged from hospital.

Until recently, mental health training in both nursing and medical curricula was largely unsatisfactory. Things have improved, but training remains predominantly hospital-based and concentrates on the 10 per cent of conditions that are treated in this setting. Very little training takes place in the community on the conditions that never reach hospital. To aggravate the situation, psychiatric services have historically been separated from general medical services and the mentally ill are often treated by different teams at different places and times. Patients who need medical treatment often have to see several doctors. The mentally ill are both stigmatized and inconvenienced. As a result of this situation, general medical staff have developed a resistance to taking responsibility for the mentally ill. The only way for any country to provide adequate treatment for psychiatric patients is to have them seen as ordinary patients within the primary care system. It is therefore vitally important to patients that all nurses have training in the diagnosis and management of mental disorders, and that clinics be adequately staffed.

Since 1994, the Mental Health Directorate (MHD) of the Gauteng Health Department has planned for the integration of mental health nursing care into primary health care in South Africa. The vision of the Directorate is to empower PHC staff to identify, manage, and/or appropriately refer the patients with mental health problems that present to their clinics. It also hopes that PHC staff will be sufficiently competent to take over the management of patients with chronic stable major mental illnesses.

The scope of mental health nursing

Over the years there has been a great deal of confusion about the role of the nurse in delivering a mental health care service on a primary health care level. It is clear that nurses on a primary health care level should be trained to do *basic screening* and basic counselling and to *identify* and *refer* patients for further assessment and management. The goal of primary health care is to assist individuals to maintain optimal health, which would reduce the need for more specialized care at the other levels. Table 1.1 outlines the scope of mental health at primary health care level. This outline provides the nurse with a structure of what is expected on this level.

Table 1.1 Scope of mental health at primary health care level

---

Service	Performance indicators
Assess and identify mental health related problems.	● Identify and handle problems needing mental health intervention timeously and appropriately before referral.
Administer emergency treatment for mental health related problems according to set protocols.	● Identify mental health emergencies and provide adequate intervention.
Provide ongoing care for chronic patients on medication within the scope of the Essential Drugs List (EDL).	● Ensure that patients are able to get their medication from the nearest clinic, as long as it is not specialist medication (i.e. restricted drugs not available at PHC level).
Do routine follow-up of stable chronically mentally ill patients and defaulters.	● Ensure that chronically mentally ill people receive routine care at the nearest clinic for their maintenance in the community.
Do home visits for mentally ill people.	● Keep a record of known mentally ill people at the clinic and include a verified psychosocial history. ● Give medication at home when patients cannot come to the clinic.
Refer patients.	● Refer patients needing more advanced care than offered at clinic level.

Table 1.1 continued

Provide basic counselling.	● Implement initial on-the-spot counselling where needed before referral for long-term counselling.
Maintain psychosocial rehabilitation of patients within the community.	● Make sure that each clinic keeps a record of patients undergoing psychosocial rehabilitation in the immediate community and develops a schedule for those interventions.
Promote health through psychoeducation.	● Plan and implement mental health campaigns in compliance with the mental health calendar. ● Establish life skills programmes in schools and youth groups. ● Provide information on mental health issues.
Undertake liaison and support.	● Liaise and collaborate with NGOs, CBOs, the private sector, traditional healers, and governmental structures in dealing with mental health issues.
Provide school health services.	● Screen and identify potential mental health problems through identification and referral of common sensory and developmental problems. ● Train teachers to identify and refer emotional and behavioural problems.

Table 1.1 continued

Provide institutional support.	• Promote healthy relationships between caregivers and children in children's homes, and identify and refer emotional/behavioural problems early. • Provide consultations, training, medical services, health inspections, and therapist support to all facilities for the mentally disabled and to psychogeriatrics in the immediate vicinity.
Promote psychoeducation programmes to combat stigma.	• Form community mental health forums and provide psychoeducation and support to families with mentally ill individuals.
Offer substance abuse services and crisis management (suicidal assessment).	• Screen and provide treatment for substance abuse related problems, as well as crisis management.
Perform forensic roles directed at managing aspects of violence within communities.	• Screen and identify survivors of violence. • Collect evidence. • Provide survivors of violence with initial counselling and proper referral.

Source: Adapted from Madela, E: 2000

Structure of mental health services

Mental health services that are to be effective and user-friendly should be within the reach of each individual. All communities, even in the most remote, underserved areas, are entitled to equal service. This can be achieved by a decentralized community-based mental health service.

Figure 1.1 Mental health services

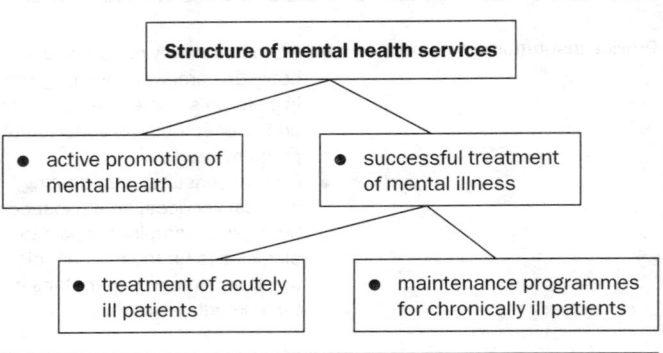

Figure 1.1 shows the areas that should receive special attention. Many psychiatric disorders have a chronic waxing and waning course. It is beneficial for both the patients and the health budget if these patients are cared for in such a way that they do not relapse.

Levels of referral

See Table 1.2 for a summary of the mental health system.

Primary care level

The majority of patients are treated at primary care level. This could be as much as 80 per cent of those who need help. Nurses should:

- be aware of and on the lookout for mental illness and should actively promote mental health;
- have the essential diagnostic and therapeutic skills for early diagnosis and intervention;
- run successful maintenance programmes for the chronically mentally ill in the community; and
- establish well-functioning consultation and referral systems.

At primary care level the consultation system should consist of:
- a 24-hour telephone consultation facility; and
- a regular on-site visit by a multi-professional psychiatric team.

Only uncomplicated work should be managed at primary care level. All complicated and therapy-resistant work should be referred to the psychiatric team because:
- nurses do not usually have sufficient training to manage these patients; and
- it can be too time-consuming for nurses and can result in overburdening and neglect of other essential work that has to be done at primary care level.

Psychoeducational groups are the best way for nurses to assist patients and their families with chronic psychiatric illness. Long-term groups for patients and their family members are the most effective and cost-effective method of treatment.

Secondary care level

A small percentage of the workload, approximately 15 to 20 per cent, is managed at the secondary level. The consultation system consists of a specialist psychiatric team responsible for:
- telephone consultations with nurses;
- on-site consultations and liaison work; and
- complicated diagnostic and therapeutic work together with therapy-resistant cases.

This level of service is an essential support system for the nurse. It is important to ensure that this support is user-friendly for nurses.

Tertiary care level

The tertiary care level of service is responsible for:
- in-service and formal training;
- research work;
- complicated and therapy-resistant work;

- management of highly specialized therapeutic programmes;
- development and implementation of special primary prevention programmes;
- development of cost-effective therapeutic programmes; and
- maintenance of an open consultation-liaison system between the three levels of care.

Nurses should find the tertiary care level supportive and user-friendly. Consultation and referral support is essential if

Table 1.2 Proposed mental health system at the district level

Level 5	
	Health worker
Tertiary level of care	Specialist regional/ tertiary hospital team
	Psychiatrists
	Psychologists
	Psychiatric nurses
	Occupational therapists
	Social workers
Level 4	
Secondary level of care	Specialist district team
	Specialist psychiatric nurse
	Psychologist
	Occupational therapist
	Social worker
	Consultant psychiatrist

nurses are to function effectively. Nurses should not be over-burdened with complicated and therapy-resistant work. At all stages, nurses should do what is best for the patient. Unnecessary referrals could be detrimental to the patient. Likewise, non-referral could be detrimental to non-responders or patients with complicated mental illnesses. Nurses must be equipped to do this risk-benefit calculation. A user-friendly consultation and referral system will make this decision a team effort and relieve the pressure on the nurse. Table 1.2 summarizes the decentralized community-based mental health service described above.

Level 5

Function

- Provide long-term in-patient care.
- Provide out-patient care.
- Provide training, support, and back-up to district teams.
- Plan and develop mental health services in the regions in conjunction with district teams.

Level 4

- Provide short-term in-patient care.
- Assess, diagnose, prescribe, revise, and initiate psychopharmacological treatment.
- Provide psychological therapy, occupational therapy, and social work services.
- Provide support and back-up to psychiatric nurses at community health centers.
- Plan and develop mental health services for the district in conjunction with psychiatric nurses in community areas.

Table 1.2 continued

Level 3	
	Psychiatric nurses
	General practitioner

Level 2	
Primary level of care	Primary health care nurses

Level 1	
	Traditional healers
	Community health workers
	Auxiliary workers
	Social workers

Level 3

- Assess, diagnose, prescribe, and initiate treatment.
- Revise treatment.
- Develop and implement community-based mental health programmes.
- Make referrals to specialists and regional hospitals.
- Train and support primary health care nurses.
- Provide counselling.
- Offer consultations.
- Implement a health information system.

Level 2

- Screen for mental health problems.
- Offer emergency treatment for mentally ill persons.
- Provide counselling.
- Make referrals to level 3.
- Offer basic rehabilitation.
- Provide psychoeducation.
- Provide follow-up medication.
- Support community health workers.

Level 1

- Promote mental health.
- Recognize mental health problems.
- Make referrals to level 2.
- Provide basic counselling.

In addition to the above functions:
- Support mentally ill persons and families.
- Provide psychoeducation.
- Offer basic rehabilitation.
- Monitor patient compliance with prescribed drug regimen.

2 Mental health versus mental illness

What is mental illness?

The brain is the organ that controls behaviour. However obvious this might seem, it cannot be overstated. The scientific view of how behaviour is regulated has two fundamental components:

- the organism with a brain; and
- the environment.

Whatever factors may have been important in the development of the individual's personality, the personality becomes relatively set and is not easily changed in adulthood. In other words, brain function becomes fairly stable and is not easily modified ('old brain'). Current reactions and experiences are important in everyday behaviour, and certainly important when people *in trouble* need help. People with *illnesses* on the other hand, constitute a different group. There may be interplay between being *in trouble* and *developing illness*. Mental illness has to do with altered physiology (function) and in some cases both the physiology and the structure of the brain are altered.

People with major psychiatric disorder have *disease* of the brain. This has become increasingly clear with improved understanding of brain function and of the techniques of measuring brain function and structure.

Causes of mental illness

Genetic factors

Genetic factors often play a part in causing mental illness and in a patient's predisposition to develop a disease. Genes play an important part in personality type. Genes are not codes of life that become dormant or are placed in cold storage after development. They are constantly involved in the dynamic control of many cell functions. So the genes are being read all the time. A large number of genes are of particular concern in the brain. The brain is under constant genetic regulation throughout life. The brain sets limitations or biases on the kind of person each of us can be. These biases seem to be set by the differences in certain systems that affect the person's emotions and behaviour. These systems are primarily genetically regulated.

Environmental factors

Environmental factors also influence the interaction and effect of these systems on behavioural responses. *Environment* refers to relatively *normal* influences. Severe stress may result in changed function of the brain. A brain injury, on the other hand, is an environmental influence that puts the whole matter into the *disease* category, since it changes both brain structure and function.

What is *normal* and what is *abnormal* is a complex subject. It is helpful to consider people in two categories, namely:

- those with brain disease; and
- those with unusual personality variations.

The first group constitutes those with brain disease associated with behaviour that is unusual or recognizable as abnormal. An example would be a schizophrenic patient who believes that *radiation* transmitters are being beamed on her to hurt her. This is unusual behaviour for her, and not within her culture. The symptoms are caused by brain disease.

The second group constitutes people who have difficulty in managing life for some reason or are unusual or troublesome to society. This is an enduring pattern of inner experience and behaviour that is related to personality. There are undoubtedly individuals who are unusual, but are able to manage life. Such individuals may have complaints, or society may complain about them. They demonstrate unusual personality variations. Some may be called *neurotic* or be referred to as having *psychopathology*. An example would be an anxious person who has always been timid and may become panicky at times and lose confidence during a period of extreme stress. This would be an exaggeration of his pre-morbid personality.

In many areas of brain dysfunction our knowledge is advancing. Obsessive-compulsive disorder was always thought to be a *neurotic* illness or anxiety disorder. New evidence of abnormal brain function and chemistry, and genetic loading is moving this condition to the *disease* category.

When evaluating ideas about a brain disorder, treatment programmes must be reproducible and testable and yield improvement rates that are not based on chance.

Good *common sense* may still go further than a narrow, highly theoretical approach that has never been tested or is untestable. In advanced training programmes nurses should critically evaluate jargon and not simply accept ill-defined processes with uncertain outcomes.

Mental health versus mental illness

Mental health is more than the absence of the symptoms of disease. Mentally healthy people:

- react adequately in terms of societal norms;
- feel comfortable about themselves;
- experience emotions freely but are not incapacitated by fear, anger, love, jealousy, guilt, and worry;
- neither under- nor over-estimate themselves;
- accept their shortcomings yet have respect for themselves;

- work productively, making use of their own capacities and putting their best efforts into whatever they are doing;
- interact well with others, give and receive love, and have satisfying and lasting personal relationships;
- respect and consider others and act responsibly towards them;
- set realistic goals, shaping their environment wherever possible and adjusting to it when necessary;
- think for themselves, accept responsibility, and make their own decisions;
- welcome new ideas and experiences;
- deal with their problems as they arise; and
- get along easily with others and are likeable.

All people become upset sometimes, for a variety of reasons. However, they know that reactions such as anxiety, anger, sadness, or confusion are normal and don't last very long. They don't consider themselves mentally ill because they feel this way. Usually they aren't disturbed by such changes in their feelings.

For example, it is natural for students to feel anxious before they write exams. In fact, anxiety may motivate them to study for, and pass, their exams. This anxiety is constructive. Only a few students become so anxious that they cannot study. These students forget what they read, cannot sleep, and may be unable to sit for their exams. This is not healthy.

Similarly, it is natural for a mother to grieve when she loses a child. She may cry frequently, lose interest in normal activities, sleep poorly, and have little appetite. Usually she will gradually reconcile herself with the loss, and begin to do her everyday work again. Only if she cannot work for many months, neglects her other children, and still struggles to sleep, would her sadness be considered abnormal.

Not all mental illness is severe and permanent. Most people accept that some sadness and anxiety are inevitable. These people are mentally healthy, with a good attitude to life, and some good relationships. Everyone has the potential to become depressed or anxious when faced with *major* stress. If the stress is prolonged and/or severe (for example, experiencing many losses, living with ongoing violence) a mentally healthy person can become mentally ill. Some people seem to be more vulnerable to becoming mentally ill. The dividing line between mental health and mental illness is not always very clear, and there is a wide range between normal and abnormal.

One way of looking at mental illness is to look at the person's *functioning* and adaptation skills in society, in their work life, social life, and in their reactions to changes. Cultural values and norms, unemployment, and the instability in society sometimes make it difficult to make judgments about a person's functioning. Always think about people in the context of the society and culture in which they live, and then assess their level of disability and the level of distress that the symptoms are causing them.

Note: For people to be considered mentally ill, their feelings and symptoms must be more severe and cause more distress than most people's and must cause disturbances at work, and in relationships. They cannot carry out their normal activities and cannot function adequately in their environment. Some or all of the functions of the mind can become disturbed with mental illness. Mental illness gives rise to behaviour that is considered abnormal in a particular society. Figure 2.1 illustrates the characteristic differences between mental health and mental illness.

Common symptoms and signs of mental illness

An understanding of signs and symptoms promotes communication and facilitates diagnosis, management of the treatment, and prognosis. When signs and symptoms occur in a recognizable pattern, the phenomenon is described as a mental disorder. This chapter identifies common symptoms and signs in psychiatric patients. (See Part III for the symptoms of specific mental health issues and disorders.)

Abnormalities of mood

Changes in mood are common symptoms of psychiatric disorders.

Figure 2.1 Characteristic differences between mental health and mental illness

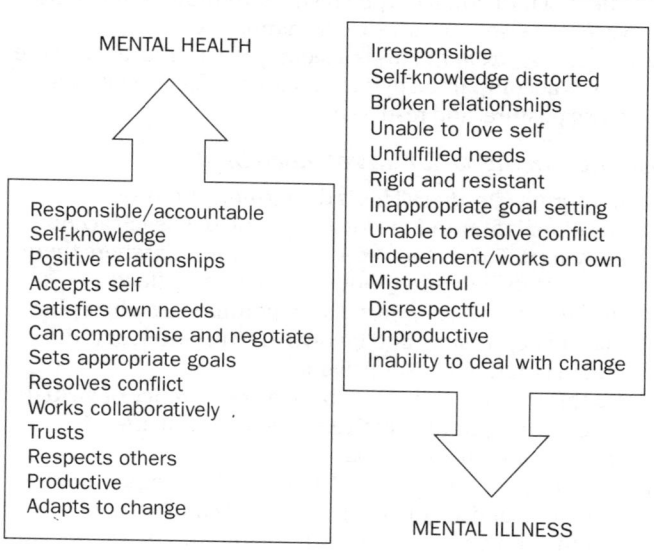

MENTAL HEALTH

Responsible/accountable
Self-knowledge
Positive relationships
Accepts self
Satisfies own needs
Can compromise and negotiate
Sets appropriate goals
Resolves conflict
Works collaboratively .
Trusts
Respects others
Productive
Adapts to change

Irresponsible
Self-knowledge distorted
Broken relationships
Unable to love self
Unfulfilled needs
Rigid and resistant
Inappropriate goal setting
Unable to resolve conflict
Independent/works on own
Mistrustful
Disrespectful
Unproductive
Inability to deal with change

MENTAL ILLNESS

The following distinctions are important:
- *mood* is a pervasive and sustained emotion, i.e. it is a subjective description of emotion as felt by the patient;
- *affect* is the observed expression of emotion; and
- *emotion* is a complexity of feelings (anger, sadness, happiness, and fear are the four primary feelings).

Changes in the nature of mood

- *Depression:* This is a feeling of sadness (mood) associated with a characteristic facial expression, body posture, and restricted gestures (affect).
- *Elation (mania):* An affect consisting of feelings of euphoria, triumph, intense self-satisfaction or optimism; it can be present in normal people.

- *Anxiety:* This is common in many mental disorders. It is a feeling of apprehension and anticipation of danger associated with a furrowed brow and tense posture. The affected individual may be restless, tremulous, and pale with increased sweating of the hands, etc.
- *Anger (Aggression):* This is a feeling of extreme displeasure that is accompanied by a characteristic facial expression, tense posture, and restlessness.

Changes in the variability of mood or affect

- *Inappropriate affect:* This is disharmony between the emotional tone and the idea, thought, or speech accompanying it. This is common in schizophrenia where there is incongruity between thoughts and mood/affect.
- *Blunted (restricted) affect:* This is common in schizophrenia and depression, and involves a diminution or reduction in emotional responsiveness.
- *Flat affect:* This is characterized by the absence or virtual absence of signs of affective expression. Flat affect is common in schizophrenia.
- *Lability:* This is exaggerated emotional responsiveness with rapid and abrupt changes. Mood can fluctuate within a short space of time – even minutes or hours.

Abnormalities of perception

- *Illusions:* An illusion is a misperception of an external stimulus, a distortion of reality. Illusions can occur when the level of sensory stimulation is reduced, when attention is not focused, when the level of consciousness is reduced (i.e. in a delirium) or when there is a strong mood state.
- *Hallucinations:* A hallucination is a perception experienced in the absence of an external stimulus, for example hearing a voice when no one is speaking. It is experienced as true and usually as coming from the outside world. There are four types of hallucination, namely:
  - auditory hallucination (hearing voices or sounds), which is common in schizophrenia and some mood disorders;
  - visual hallucination (seeing things), which is common in substance abuse and organic brain syndromes;

- tactile hallucination (feelings things), which is common in tempral lobe epilepsy; and
- smell or taste hallucinations, which are also common in epilepsy.

Disorders of thinking – thought disorder

Disorders of the stream of thought

These disorders affect both the amount and the speed of thoughts. These disorders are characterized by:

- pressure, where thoughts are rapid, abundant, and varied;
- poverty, where thoughts are slow, few, and unvaried; and
- thought blocking, where the mind is suddenly empty and the patient loses track of his or her own thoughts.

Disorders of form of thought

Disorders of form of thought constitute a change in the way in which thoughts are linked together. It is often difficult to understand the patient. These disorders are characterized by:

- flight of ideas (rapid movement from one topic to another with linkage between the different topics);
- perseveration (persistent and inappropriate repetition of the same sequence of thoughts/words); and
- loosening of association (a lack of logical connection between parts of a train of thought, where there is no linkage and thoughts jump from one topic to another).

Delusion

A delusion is a false personal belief that cannot be changed by rational argument or evidence and is not in keeping with the person's level of education or cultural background. Delusions are common in depression and schizophrenia.

A *primary delusion* occurs suddenly without an identifiable mental event leading up to it and is fully developed. A *secondary delusion* arises from a preceding experience and is inclined to 'grow'. The following are common delusional themes:

- persecutory (paranoid);
- grandiose and expansive;
- guilt and worthlessness;

- jealousy;
- sexual or amorous;
- hypochondriacal;
- nihilistic;
- religious;
- delusions of control; and
- delusions of reference.

A *mood-congruent delusion* is a delusion that is consistent with the mood: for example, death or paranoia, and depression. Mood-congruent delusions are common in mood disorders. A mood-incongruent delusion is a delusion that is inconsistent with mood. Mood-incongruent delusions are common in schizophrenia. For example, a homeless person believes that he or she is a millionaire.

An *overvalued idea* is an isolated preoccupying and strongly held belief that dominates a person's life and may affect his or her actions but (unlike a delusion) has been derived through normal mental processes. The idea can be changed by confronting reality (unlike a delusion, which is fixed).

Obsessive and compulsive symptoms

Obsessions

Obsessions are recurrent persistent 'senseless' ideas, thoughts, images, or impulses that are ego-dystonic (uncomfortable), that is they are not experienced as voluntarily produced, but rather as ideas that invade consciousness. The characteristic feature is the subjective sense of struggle (resistance) against the intruding mental phenomena. Obsessional symptoms include:

- thoughts;
- ruminations (thoughts that recur continuously);
- doubts;
- impulses; and
- phobias.

Common obsessional themes are dirt and contamination (dirty hands), aggressive action (harm somebody), orderliness (arranging objects), illness (idea of cancer), sex (disgusting thoughts), and religion (blasphemous thoughts).

Compulsions

Compulsions are repeated, stereotyped, and seemingly purposeful actions that the person feels compelled to carry out while realizing that they are irrational (compulsive rituals). The goal of compulsions is to prevent or reduce anxiety or distress or to prevent some future event from occurring and not to provide pleasure or gratification. Compulsive symptoms include:

- checking;
- cleaning, e.g. washing hands;
- counting; and
- dressing.

Phobias

A phobia is a persistent, irrational, exaggerated, pathological dread (fear) of a specific stimulus or situation, which results in a compelling desire to avoid the feared stimulus. Phobias include:

- social phobia, which is a dread of public humiliation, and of speaking, performing, or eating in public;
- specific phobias, e.g. for spiders or snakes; and
- numerous other phobias, such as agoraphobia and claustrophobia.

Depersonalization and derealization

Depersonalization is the experience of feeling unreal, detached, and unable to feel emotion (the self is foreign). Derealization is an experience where the environment feels unreal and other people seem lifeless (the environment is strange). These two symptoms can occur in healthy people, but also in anxiety disorders, depressive disorders, schizophrenia, and temporal lobe epilepsy.

Motor symptoms and signs

Abnormalities of facial expression, posture, and social behaviour are common in mental disorders of all kinds. Two classic motor disturbances in catatonic schizophrenia are:

- stupor, where the individual is immobile, mute, and unresponsive; and
- excitement, i.e. uncontrolled motor activity.

Memory disorders

There are different types of memory, namely:
- immediate (seconds to minutes);
- recent (past few days); and
- remote (distant past).

Amnesia

Amnesia involves partial or total inability to recall past experiences. There are two kinds of amnesia, namely:
- anterograde amnesia (after a certain point in time);and
- retrograde amnesia (before a certain point in time).

Paramnesia

Paramnesia involves falsification of memory by distortion of recall. There are three kinds of paramnesia, namely:
- confabulation (filling of gaps in memory), which is common in alcohol-induced amnesia;
- déja vu (a feeling of familiarity), which is common in temporal lobe epilepsy; and
- jamais vu (a feeling of strangeness), which is also common in temporal lobe epilepsy.

Disorders of consciousness

Consciousness is awareness of the self and the environment. Disorders include:
- *Disorientation:* Orientation is disturbed in terms of time, place, and person.
- *Clouding of consciousness:* This condition manifests as drowsiness, impaired attention, concentration and memory, and slow, muddled thinking.
- *Stupor:* The patient is mute, immobile, and unresponsive but has his or her eyes open, sees objects, and follows movement.
- *Delirium:* The patient is bewildered, restless, confused, disoriented, and fearful, and has hallucinations.
- *Coma:* This is a profound degree of unconsciousness.

Disturbances of intellectual function

Intelligence is the ability to understand, recall, mobilize, and integrate previous experiences in meeting new situations.

- *Mental challenge (handicap):* This is a lack of intelligence and can be classified as mild, moderate, severe, or profound.
- *Dementia:* This is organic and global deterioration of intellectual functioning without clouding of consciousness.
- *Pseudodementia:* This includes features of dementia that are not caused by 'organic' deterioration of the brain (for example, depression).

Disorders of attention and concentration

Attention is the ability to focus on an activity (deficits are common in children). Concentration is the ability to maintain focus. Many kinds of psychiatric disorders can impair attention and concentration, but particularly anxiety disorder, depressive disorder, mania, schizophrenia, and organic disorder.

Insight

Basically, insight implies an accurate awareness of one's own mental condition. Lack of insight implies that an individual is not fully aware of his or her own mental condition or the need for treatment. This situation is common in psychotic disorders.

Judgement

Judgement is the ability to evaluate external events correctly and includes the individual's response to external events.

Although the nurse needs to elicit details on the signs and symptoms of mental disorder one should never lose sight of the patient as a person. The nurse must take particular care in eliciting symptoms and signs when he or she is communicating with the patient via a translator. The translator should give the nurse a verbatim or word-for-word translation. This is particularly important when signs of thought disorder are being elicited.

3 Mental health and mental illness in an African context

African concepts of health and sickness have traditionally been attributed to causes outside of the patient. Illness may be caused by evil spirits, evil objects, or an evil person. It may be due to visitations of ancestors or gods, or the illness may be a call from the ancestors to become a *sangoma* (diviner-healer). Illness is seldom attributed simply to some physical disorder or malfunction of the body itself.

When patients and their families seek help, they will ask who has caused the illness and why. Attention is focused on some person or object, or on the appeasement of gods. Ancestors might have been displeased by some act or by omission of rites that either propitiate or appease the spirits.

In some cases the patient may be revered as representing the embodiment of the spirits or ancestors. This depends on the belief system of the patient and the community. Seeking a cure for an illness is sometimes regarded as interference that may anger the spirit.

For the various presentations of mental and physical illness, a *sangoma* or other diviner will by divination reveal what has entered the patient and what is expected to be done to rectify whatever is wrong. Some ritual or sacrifice may be prescribed: perhaps slaughtering an ox or a chicken to use entrails, skin, or feathers in a specific manner.

Should the presentation be attributable to sorcery and witchcraft, the sangoma may provide protection with medicines or may be in a position to point out the person responsible. In extreme cases, the suspect is eliminated by ritual murder.

Broadly speaking, traditional African thought concedes the presence of aberrant behaviour, which may be beyond the accepted bounds of normality. There are certain broad categories that indicate the recognition of unusual behaviour, but it is often difficult for community members to accept that the *different* behaviour is an illness. The known broad categories that describe behaviour roughly approximate some psychiatric diagnoses, but are probably best translated as *mad* or *mixed up*. In African languages there are no words to describe mental symptoms like hallucinations or delusions. Mental illnesses don't have specific names such as schizophrenia, or bipolar disorder; by contrast, physical illnesses such as tonsillitis, tuberculosis, and syphilis do have actual names.

The general absence of a concept of mental illness may explain part of the problem of providing psychiatric services in African society. The patient is not regarded as being ill and is not thought to have any need to see a doctor unless there are physical symptoms. A psychiatric diagnosis makes for a confusion of paradigms in the African setting.

In practice however, communities are increasingly seeking medical help for mental illness when they recognize that the client's behaviour is something other than expected presentations such as visits by the ancestors, bewitchment, or some other culturally recognized condition. At times patients are brought in for medical attention because their behaviour is uncontrollable or destructive. Often, the psychiatric consultation will occur only after the patient has been to numerous *sangomas* and a variety of other healers. Coming for medical help is a measure of desperation rather than acceptance that the behaviour is caused by illness. After psychiatric treatment the patient will often have a need to return for traditional *holistic* treatment and will discontinue Western medicines.

To diagnose and manage the mentally ill, practitioners trained in Western medicine need to know the cultural attitudes of their patients and will have to consult experts. Beliefs may vary greatly between tribes and also between clans within tribes. Religions will have their own variations that will require investigation.

A practitioner who is working in an unfamiliar cultural setting and needs to distinguish between mental health and mental illness must find answers to the following questions:

- Is the patient 'sick'?
- Does the patient function normally within the culture in terms of occupation, social interaction, and self-care?

Good collateral information from members of the family and community is essential if these questions are to be answered.

In treating the patient, the best results will be obtained when dissonance, i.e. lack of agreement between Western medical intervention and the patient's world-view are kept to a minimum. This means working closely with the patient's family and community support system.

Cultural syndromes

Comparative psychiatry uses formal epidemiological or less formal observational and clinical methods to describe and analyse cultural variations in the incidence or prevalence of syndromes and symptoms.

Comparative psychiatry is difficult under the best of circumstances. The major psychiatric symptoms and symptom clusters, including those at the core of the major disorders appear to manifest themselves in all societies. These symptoms include anxiety, mania, depression, suicidal ideation, thought disorder, paranoia, and somatization disorder. These disorders frequently manifest themselves as folk illnesses, with labels that subdivide the range of symptom patterns differently from labels given by Western psychiatrists and psychologists.

Some cultures may refrain from labelling but nevertheless recognize the abnormality, and even its treatability. Many give labels that are surprisingly close to the cross-national comparisons of Western psychiatric diagnoses.

The African concept of mental illness

A clear understanding of African culture-bound syndromes (CBS) depends on a clear understanding of African concepts of mental illness.

In the past, the universal belief in supernatural phenomena influenced concepts of the causes of mental illness; specifically the influence of witchcraft and the spirits of the ancestors. Medicine that relies primarily on science is a new concept. Cultures differ in their definitions of health, illness, and healing.

African concepts of mental illness encompass many systems such as ancestors, folk beliefs, and witchcraft; and accommodate modern medical science without difficulty. All the systems function simultaneously within the African culture and within the individual and easily fit into and complement one another.

In terms of the African concept of mental illness, the causes of mental illness can be broadly divided into three groups.

Biological causes

When the cause is biological it manifests itself as:

- illness as a malfunction of the brain due to injury or toxins, for example alcohol or dagga; or
- a hereditary illness (*ufuzo*) – diseases that are believed to run in families, for example epilepsy, mental handicap, and schizophrenia.

Psychological causes

Psychological causes for illness would include maternal deprivation. There is an African saying *Intandane entle wumokhothwa ngunina*, which means 'a good orphan is he who is loved by the mother', which emphasizes the importance of a good mother-child relationship.

Illness is never attributed entirely to biological or psychological factors. The question *who*, or *what* made *me* sick remains. Often, the only answer that may be accepted is that *someone or something* has caused the illness.

Socio-cultural causes

The four major influences in African culture-bound syndromes are:

- ancestors;
- witches and witchcraft;
- other spirits; and
- dreams.

Ancestors and illness

The ancestors are the departed dead of up to five generations. They are in a state of personal immortality and the process of dying is not yet complete. They are the custodians of family affairs, traditions, ethics, and activities.

Offence in these areas is ultimately an offence against the ancestors. Failure to placate and pacify the ancestors leads to misfortune and illness. Even though ancestors cannot perform miracles, people experience a sense of psychological relief when they pour out their hearts and lay their troubles before their seniors who know their needs and simultaneously have full access to the channels of direct communication with God.

Witchcraft

Some African people feel and believe that the various illnesses, misfortunes, and accidents that they encounter and experience are caused by the use of this mystical power in the hands of a *mthakathi* (witch or wizard). For many African people, diseases are not purely physical experiences: they are mystical experiences. People in the village will talk freely about these mystical experiences because, regardless of what scientists might say, these experiences are part of their personal world of reality. Nothing harmful happens by chance. Everything is caused by *someone*, either directly or through the use of mystical powers or witchcraft.

Other spirits

According to traditional African belief, a person consists of a body and a spirit that are joined in a living person. The spirit becomes part of the body during conception and leaves the body during death. The spirit does not lose its identity but is believed to linger around the body after death. People will still have conversations with and visions of the dead and are not necessarily psychotic when having these conversations.

Dreams

According to traditional belief, people may also encounter the spirits of the living dead through dreams and visions. During this process they talk to the spirits and receive instructions or requests from them. Demands made by them are usually fulfilled. Other methods of satisfying the ancestors include seeking the help of traditional healers or diviners (Mbiti, 1991). Nurses should be culturally sensitive and aware of the impact of beliefs. They should not misdiagnose patients who follow cultural traditions.

Culture-bound syndromes

Culture-bound syndromes are recurrent, locality-specific patterns of aberrant behaviour and troubling experiences that may or may not be linked to a particular recognized diagnostic category in Western terms.

Many of these patterns are indigenously considered to be *illnesses*, or at least afflictions, and most have local names. Although presentations conforming to the major DSM-IV categories can be found throughout the world, local cultural factors influence the particular symptoms, course, and social response. In contrast to the illnesses described in DSM-IV, culture-bound syndromes are generally limited to specific societies or cultural areas. They are arranged into localized, folk-diagnostic categories, which provide frameworks that offer coherent meaning for certain repetitive, patterned, and troubling sets of experiences and observations.

The cross-cultural distribution of some disorders is so skewed that the differences can probably be accepted without any strictly reliable epidemiological methods whatever. A specific disorder may have a label, social construction, explanation, or mental content that is culturally unique, and is also bound to its cultural meaning to the extent that essentially it would not exist (or would be something else) in the absence of that particular framework.

Culture-bound syndromes rarely fit neatly into accepted diagnostic entities. Aberrant behaviour that a diagnostician using DSM-IV may divide into several categories may be included in a single folk category. In contrast, presentations that a diagnostician using DSM-IV may regard as belonging to a single category may be divided into several categories by an indigenous clinician. By comparison, some conditions have been conceptualized as culture-bound syndromes specific to industrialized culture (e.g. anorexia nervosa, dissociative identity disorder) given their apparent rarity or absence in other cultures. Note that all industrialized societies include distinctive subcultures and widely diverse immigrant groups who may present with disorders.

Characteristics of culture-bound syndromes

Culture-bound syndromes are not homogenous, in terms of either their symptomatology or their aetiology. However, they do have the following common elements:

- Patients are generally normal before the onset of the syndrome.
- Their behaviour is usually some kind of acting out that attracts attention.
- The trigger for their behaviour may be difficult to isolate but is usually some psychosocial stressor.
- There is no adequate information available on the pre-morbid personalities of these patients. Labelling them *histrionic personalities* without sound evidence is not justified.
- These illnesses do not generally involve any deterioration in personality or functioning.
- These patients are usually young females.
- There is no evidence of an underlying functional psychosis.
- The illnesses may be either isolated occurrences or they may be chronic.
- The illnesses are always attributed to an outside force.
- Somatic symptoms predominate.

- Amnesia is almost always present.
- Illnesses may improve spontaneously or may require treatment with benzodiazepines or antipsychotics for a period.
- Therapy should be multi-disciplinary and take account of the patient's culture.

The African culture-bound syndromes

A number of African culture-bound syndromes have been described; but for the purpose of this book only two will be considered.

The Fufunyane Syndrome (Amafufunyane)

This is a condition little known outside southern Africa. A number of South African researchers have contributed towards the understanding of this syndrome. Various authors have described the following signs and symptoms:

- children sometimes affected;
- mass manifestations or epidemics;
- sudden onset;
- voices of the opposite sex;
- hysterical and aggressive behaviour;
- agitation;
- xeroglosia;
- suicide threats;
- altered state of consciousness;
- amnesia;
- listlessness;
- loss of appetite;
- stress;
- depression; and
- anxiety.

Other descriptions omit some of the symptoms and add:

- amnesia;
- fear of witchcraft;
- throwing themselves about;
- tearing their clothes; and °
- somatic symptoms such as abdominal pain, headaches, body cramps, and signs that would fit the dissociative

trance state listed in the DSM-IV. There seem to be core symptoms, but there is wide variability with time and place.

The Fufunyane Syndrome manifests some features of a panic attack, namely:

- palpitations;
- pounding heart or accelerated heart rate;
- sweating;
- trembling;
- shaking;
- smothering;
- shortness of breath;
- feeling of choking;
- chest pain or discomfort;
- nausea and abdominal distress;
- dizziness;
- unsteadiness;
- lightheadedness;
- faintness;
- derealization;
- depersonalization;
- fear of losing control;
- fear of going crazy;
- fear of dying;
- paraesthesia; and
- chills or hot flushes.

Following the attack of Fufunyane the patient returns to completely normal function but usually has amnesia for the event.

There are similarities between Fufunyane and Ataque de Nervios, which is a condition principally reported among Latin-American and Latin-Mediterranean groups in the Caribbean.

The Thwasa Syndrome (Ukuthwasa)

This is culturally regarded as an acceptable form of ancestral spirit possession when a person is called to become an *inyanga* or *sangoma* (traditional healer: herbalist and diviner).

The symptoms vary and may manifest as anything from anxiety or depression to actual physical illness. These individuals may also mimic schizophrenia or schizophreniform disorder but they are highly functional people and remain so once the symptoms have abated. A *sangoma* or an *inyanga* diagnoses this syndrome. Dreams play an important role in the symptomatology of this condition. These are vivid dreams, which at times may appear hallucinatory. They enormously influence the behaviour of these patients because the reality in dreams is equated with reality experienced during waking hours.

The symptoms will only be cured by undergoing training as an *inyanga* or *sangoma*. This would be similar to medical school training; but there is no set curriculum or number of years in training. It all depends on how the ancestors guide the individual during the training. It takes between two and ten years, and as in medical schools, some never qualify, but will remain at medical school as technicians under authority. Those who qualify set up their own practices and, just as in Western medicine, there are good ones and bad ones.

Guidelines for a culture-congruent approach

The nurse should bear in mind the following guidelines (Madela-Mntla, *et al*: 1999).

Assessment

During the assessment phase the nurse should ask the patient the following questions to determine the onset of the illness, the cause, and treatment:

- What do you call your problem?
- What do you think caused it?
- Why do you think it started when it did?
- What does your sickness do to you? How does it work?
- How severe is your sickness? Will it have a long or a short duration?
- What kind of treatment do you think you should receive?

The nurse must also use additional information such as a history from those who know the psychiatric patient and information already available in the clinical documents to gain a clear understanding of the patient's views.

During this phase of assessment the nurse must:

- Encourage psychiatric patients to express themselves;
- Show acceptance, respect, and understanding of the psychiatric patient's perspective.
- Listen actively while patients air their views.
- Treat patients as equals.
- Share his or her own perspectives on the patient's mental illness (by giving responses to questions asked by the patient).
- Encourage the patient also to listen to the nurse's perspective, and attempt to teach patients through this process.
- Focus the patient's attention on the common goal, namely to promote, maintain, and restore mental health.

Planning

The nurse and the psychiatric patient must also negotiate a treatment plan that they will follow. At the planning stage, the following should be attended to:

- The nurse must inform the patient of his or her own perspective of the psychiatric treatment.
- The nurse must negotiate a compromise between his or her view and those of the patient on the psychiatric treatment.
- The nurse must plan with the patient the best treatment for the mental illness.
- The PHC treatment plan must take into consideration the cultural beliefs, values, and practices of the patient and the nurse.

Implementation

At the implementation stage the nurse and the psychiatric patient take action to apply the agreed treatment plan. The guidelines at this stage involve the following strategies and attitudes:

- Both the nurse and the psychiatric patient must adhere to the treatment plan agreed upon during negotiation.

- The nurse must encourage the positive behaviours of the patient.
- The nurse must support and assist patients to enable them to mobilize resources in their internal and external environments.
- The nurse must discourage health practices that are harmful and must encourage those that are helpful or neutral.
- The nurse must continuously give patients feedback about their progress.
- The nurse must liaise with other health professionals and with the patient's family.

Evaluation

The evaluation stage involves assessing whether the objectives set at the beginning of treatment have been achieved. At this stage, the nurse must:

- observe signs of cultural care maintenance, accommodation, and restructuring; and
- evaluate the patient's ability to mobilize resources in his or her internal and external environments.

Evaluation should:

- take place throughout the process (along with negotiations);
- serve as the basis for reassessment; and
- aim to determine whether treatment has succeeded in promoting, maintaining, and restoring the client's mental health.

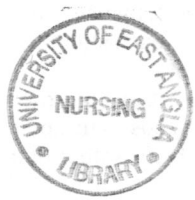

4 The nursing process

The nurse should view each patient as a whole person and understand that mental illness emerges out of the interaction of biological, cultural, psychological, and social factors. Good health encompasses the physical, mental, and spiritual aspects together.

The South African Nursing Council clearly states that nurses should use the scientific method in nursing, called *the nursing process*. The nursing process is a special way of thinking and acting:

- It is a systematic, problem-solving approach used to identify, prevent, and treat actual or potential mental health problems, and to promote mental health.
- It provides a framework in which nurses can use their critical and analytical thinking skills to express human caring and assist patients in meeting their health needs.
- It gives clear direction for planning, implementing, and evaluating effective, individualized nursing care, usually in the form of a written nursing care plan.
- It focuses on the patient, and encourages patient input at each step.

To promote mental health in an integrated way, the nurse needs to understand and apply both the basic principles and the five steps of the nursing process.

The five steps of the nursing process

The nursing process consists of five interrelated steps, namely:
- assessment;
- diagnosis;
- planning;
- implementation; and
- evaluation.

Step 1: Assessment

The assessment is the first step of the process. To perform an assessment, the nurse has to collect, validate, organize, and record data using interview, observation, and examination techniques. Nurses should:
- apply critical-thinking skills, using the appropriate theoretical knowledge, and demonstrating an awareness of ethical issues such as confidentiality and honesty;
- use directive and non-directive interviewing techniques, adapting them to the special needs of the patient (assessment interviewing skills);
- collect and organize data according to various conceptual models such as Maslow's Hierarchy of Needs, Roy's Adaptation Theory, Peplau's Interpersonal Theory, and Nursing Theory for Health promotion (see case study in Step 2); and
- consider the moral principles of autonomy (the patient retains ultimate responsibility).

Guidelines for assessment

The following are key guidelines for conducting an assessment interview:

Collect data

- Collect *subjective* data. This should include a mental state examination and/or a mini-mental state examination following the guidelines in Chapters 9 and 19.
- Collect *objective* data by performing a physical examination to review the body systems and vital signs.

Validate data with patient
- Compare subjective and objective data.
- Validate conflicting data.

Organize and record data
- Initial assessment: Use printed form (Table 4.1).
- Ongoing assessment: Keep nursing progress notes.

Table 4.1 Areas to include in a complete nursing assessment

Psychosocial factors	Notes
● Identifying data	
Name	
Address	
Birth	
Marital status	
Sex	
Race	
● Presenting data	
Nature of the problem	
Time of occurrence	
Reason for seeking care at this time	
● Family information	
Family's generational structure	
Home environment	
Physical and mental health	
Financial status	
Developmental stage in family life cycle	
Family structure	
Intra-family relationships	
Socio-cultural family content	
Strengths and weaknesses	
Identified problem	

Communication patterns	
Interaction patterns	
Crisis response	
● Socio-economic status	
Occupation	
Education	
Leisure time	
Residence	
Income	
● Life values	
Ethnicity/culture	
Religious behaviour/spirituality	
Beliefs about illness	
Attitudes towards life	
Living standards and self-care behaviour	
● Social habits	
Eating	
Drinking	
Drug use	
Hygiene	
● Sexual behaviour	
Preference	
Sex role	
Sex activity	
● Cognition	
Consciousness	
Orientation	Perform a mental state examination (MSE) and a mini-mental state examination (MMSE). See Chapters 9 and 19
Attention	
Perception	
Apperception	
Thought content	
Thought form	
Thought progress	
Memory	
Self-concept	
Body image	

● Affect	
Depersonalization	
Continuum of despair to ecstasy	
Affective ambivalence	MSE + MMSE
Inadequate affect	
Inappropriate affect	
Anxiety	
● Volition (observed)	
Appearance	
Motor activity	
Communication	
Social support	
Size of social network	
Intensity, durability, multidimensionality, dispersion, and frequency of social linkages	
Normative context of the relationships	
Social roles	
Support available to meet role obligations during illness	
Patterns of social affiliation	
Need for social affiliation	
Medication	
Psychiatric medication	
Prescription (non-psychiatric) medication	
Over-the-counter (non-prescribed) medication	
Alcohol and street drugs	
Physiological factors	
● Medical history	
Development	
Past illnesses and injuries	
Hospitalizations	
Family history	
● Physiological status	
Body systems	
Present illnesses	
Medications and ongoing treatment	
● Health maintenance	
Health goals	

Step 2: Data base and diagnosis

During diagnosis, the second step of the nursing process, nurses apply their critical thinking skills to interpret patient data by for example, making inferences, analysing, and synthesizing data. Data is interpreted in order to identify patient health status (e.g. strengths, problems, and causes of the problems). Strengths and problems are verified with the patient, formally diagnosed (DSM-IV diagnoses), and recorded on the patient's care plan.

The following case study will help to illustrate the formulation of nursing diagnoses, and treatment goals and objectives:

Kedi Dlamini is a 36-year-old man who was admitted to a secured male ward as a Section 9 patient (compulsory admission). In desperation, his wife had him certified because he refused admission. She was afraid that he would commit suicide while at home. She described him as 'very distressed' and stated that he wasn't sleeping well. When he did manage to fall asleep, he would wake in the middle of the night, screaming and sweating. He became quite aggressive when asked about this.

Mr. Dlamini is a security guard working in a high-crime area. In the period before his admission, he had seen many of his colleagues die violently. He stated that he felt helpless. A few weeks before admission, Kedi and his partner, James Moloto, were transporting money between two banks when James was pulled from the car by a gang, who hijacked their vehicle. James was killed when one of the hijackers shot and injured him fatally. Kedi was helpless to stop James's murder.

Kedi's wife realized that he was becoming increasingly restless and irritated and talked frequently about his disappointment at the rising crime and lack of law and order in the country. He felt that violence was increasing all the time. Until his admission, Kedi was still working, but his friends and colleagues could see that he was not functioning as usual. When he witnessed violence on television, he would perspire and become highly anxious. He seemed very quiet and withdrawn and his marriage and other relationships were beginning to fail. He also talked about there being no future for him and his family. This, together with the fact that he had lost a tremendous amount of weight over the preceding month, forced his wife to seek help urgently.

Before formulating the nursing diagnosis, the nurse should first create a database of the patient's history. The database records the psychiatric symptoms.

Database of Kedi Dlamini

The key symptoms are:
- suicidal ideation;
- depressed mood and helplessness;
- poor sleep – intermittent insomnia;
- nightmares;
- sweating;
- anger – becomes aggressive;
- guilt-feelings;
- restlessness and irritability;
- decreased occupational functioning;
- hypervigilance;
- withdrawal and quietness;
- feeling that life has no meaning; and
- anorexia (weight loss).

Format for writing the nursing diagnosis

The nursing diagnosis is a statement that describes the patient's problem and related risk factors. The basic components of a nursing diagnosis are the *problem* and the *aetiology*.

Problem
- The problem part of the statement describes the patient's health state clearly and concisely.
- It identifies what should be changed about the patient's status, and it should therefore suggest a patient goal.

Aetiology
- The aetiology describes factors causing or contributing to actual problems. For potential problems, it describes the risk factors that are present.

- The aetiology enables one to individualize nursing care for a patient.

Referring to the case study, it is clear that Kedi Dlamini suffers from a high degree of emotional and mental distress (he shows the signs and symptoms of anxiety and depression). He is unable to cope with this. The aetiology could thus be described as the inability to deal with the effects of the emotional/mental trauma (namely, a brutal murder and hijacking). The nursing diagnosis would look as follows:

Figure 4.1 The nursing diagnosis

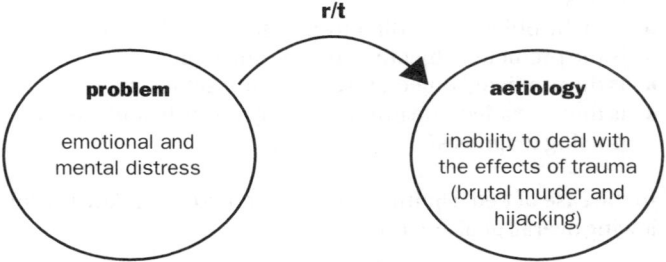

r/t

problem

emotional and mental distress

aetiology

inability to deal with the effects of trauma (brutal murder and hijacking)

The symbol r/t ('related to') connects the two main parts of the statement.

Step 3 : Planning

Patient goals and objectives

The nurse needs to formulate one overall goal and break it down into a few SMART objectives (objectives that are specific, measurable, attainable, realistic, and time-based). Note that:
- the goal is based on the problem; and
- the objectives should refer back to the patient database.

Goal

Ask these questions when formulating the goal:
- Is the goal derived from only one nursing diagnosis?

- Does the goal clearly demonstrate a satisfactory resolution of the problem?
- Is the goal appropriate to the nursing diagnosis?
- Does the goal have all the necessary components, namely subject, action, performance criteria, special conditions, and target time?
- Is the goal congruent with the total treatment plan?
- Is the goal concise?

Objectives

Ask the following questions when breaking down the overall goal into objectives:

- When possible, is the predicted objective stated in positive terms?
- Can the objective be directly measured or observed?
- Is the predicted objective specific and concrete?
- Is the predicted objective realistic and achievable?
- Is there an adequate number of objectives to address each nursing diagnosis?

In the case of Kedi Dlamini, the nurse could formulate the following overall goal and objectives:

Table 4.2 Goal and objectives for Kedi Dlamini

Goal

Relief of emotional and mental distress within the next 4 to 6 weeks.

Objectives

This will be achieved by:

- improving sleep to 6 to 8 hours per night;
- developing the ability to verbalize and deal with anxiety, anger, help-lessness, and guilt in 2 to 4 weeks, within an established nurse-patient relationship;
- providing evidence of stabilized mood (patient is able to verbalize a renewed interest in life) within 4 to 6 weeks; and
- gaining weight at a rate of 0,5 to 1 kg per week until target weight is reached.

Step 4: Implementing nursing actions

Note that nursing actions should address each set objective and should answer the following questions: Why? How? What? When? Who? The answers to these questions provide the *rationale* or reason for the action. The following are guidelines for successfully implementing the goal and objectives.

Prepare the nurse

- Determine whether you need help to perform the action safely and minimize stress to the patient.
- Be sure you know the rationale for the intervention, as well as any potential side effects or complications. When actions are based on experience in practice, examine them critically.
- Question any actions you do not understand or that seem inappropriate or potentially unsafe.
- Determine feedback points and assess the patient's response during the activity.
- Schedule activities to allow adequate time for completion.
- Delegate interventions to other team members in order to use your time efficiently.
- Improve your knowledge base by continually seeking new information.

Prepare the patient

- Determine that the action is still necessary and appropriate.
- Assess patient readiness.
- Inform the patient of what to expect and what you expect.
- Provide for privacy and comfort.

During implementation

- Adapt interventions to the individual's age, values, culture, norms, and health status.
- Encourage the patient to participate actively and responsibly.
- Perform interventions carefully and accurately and remember the target dates.
- Follow a holistic approach in setting actions for the patient, i.e. consider the physical, emotional, social, intellectual, and spiritual dimensions.

Table 4.3 illustrates the nursing actions that could be set for Kedi Dlamini. Remember to use a holistic approach that addresses all dimensions, as shown below.

Table 4.3 Nursing actions for Kedi Dlamini

Action	Rationale
Physical Dimension	
Provide recreational and diversional activities such as swimming, jogging, walking, running errands, and performing simple tasks and repetitive activities.	● Use the energy activated by anxiety to reduce anxiety and to decrease time available for introspection and preoccupation.
Promote sleep with comfort measures (warm bath, music, back rub, quiet presence of a significant person).	● Assist Kedi to relax and obtain restful sleep.
Emotional Dimension	
Facilitate the expression of feelings of anxiety by listening actively, showing respect, and expressing empathy.	● Help Kedi to assess his level of anxiety and the possible causes, and to set priorities for care. Talking about anxious feelings with another person diminishes the intensity of anxiety.
Assist Kedi in identifying subjective experience of sadness, anger, or hostility.	● Increase his awareness of feelings and plan interventions.
Explore with Kedi those situations that precipitate feelings of sadness, anger, or hostility.	● Identify causes of sadness, anger, and hostility.
Jointly develop alternatives that reduce feelings of anger, hostility, and sadness and decide on ways to implement those strategies.	● Involve Kedi in plans for treatment and promote feelings of control over life.

Table 4.3 continued

Respond warmly and empathically and convey a hopeful attitude.	• Convey understanding and confidence that Kedi can feel better.
Observe Kedi for changes in depression that indicate increased suicidal potential.	• Revise treatment goals and plan interventions.
Explore Kedi's ambivalence about life.	• Focus on positive factors that promote his will to live.

Intellectual Dimension

Speak slowly and calmly.	• Convey a relaxed attitude by using self therapeutically.
Use simple, short sentences.	• Help Kedi understand the message. Anxious patients have difficulty concentrating and processing information.
Give brief, concise directions.	• Facilitate understanding.
Refrain from making demands on, or requiring decisions from, Kedi.	• Lessen the stress and tension associated with making decisions.
Enforce rules consistently.	• Promote security – uncertainty and inconsistency create anxiety.

Social Dimension

Stay with Kedi.	• Indicate that help is available.
Remove excessive stimulation.	• Calm or relax Kedi.
Provide a safe environment with prompt attention to requests.	• Increase trust and safety, both physical and emotional.
Limit contact with others (for example, other patients or family members who are anxious).	• Prevent feelings of anxiety from being transferred to Kedi.

Table 4.3 continued

Explore secondary gains Kedi may be receiving from others through his anxious behaviour.	• Prevent him from receiving benefits and satisfaction from anxious behaviour.
If Kedi is unemployed or relocated because of anxiety problems, refer to a social worker for services.	• Initiate rehabilitation and prevent incapacitation.
Spiritual Dimension	
Refrain from discussion of beliefs and values that require decisions, until anxiety decreases.	• Prevent escalation of anxiety when issues are emotionally charged.
Help Kedi add peace and contentment to life by increasing his confidence in himself and his abilities.	• Add quality to his life without excessive anxiety.
Help Kedi see anxiety as a challenge and an opportunity to find meaning in life by emphasizing opportunities for growth instead of focusing on problems.	• Help him to master anxiety, learn problem-solving skills, improve self-esteem and develop autonomy.
Provide opportunities for Kedi to help others to gain self-satisfaction, increase self-esteem, and enrich life.	• Helping others promotes a sense of satisfaction with oneself, increases self-esteem, and enriches quality of life – one's own and others'.

Step 5: Evaluation

The nurse needs to evaluate goal achievement within a set timeframe and revise the care plan as needed.

5 Stress and mental illness

Stress is a commonly used word. We live in a stressful society. Stress is not usually defined by what causes it but by an individual's reaction to the stressor. Stress is not necessarily a nervous reaction. Brain and body are closely interrelated and stress can manifest itself in the body's reaction without conscious awareness. Stress is the reaction of the mind/brain and body to change.

The range of reactions is wide and many individuals do not find them unpleasant even though a significant degree of change may be involved. The key difference between healthy and harmful stress is that:

- healthy stress involves rapid compensation for change; but
- harmful stress results in little or no adjustment.

What is stressful for one person may not be stressful for another, and what is stressful for a person at a particular time may not be stressful for the same person at another time. Stress can be viewed as the balance between the external demands (stressor) on an individual and that individual's capacity to cope with those demands at any given time. A person's stress level can be reduced in one of two ways:

- decrease the severity of external stressors; or
- increase the ability to cope (compensate).

As Figure 5.1 shows, the combination of environmental and individual factors determines the severity of reactions to stress. While the overall responses are mediated by the hypothalamic-pituitary axis, the body's healthy reactions to stress are largely controlled by the autonomic nervous system. Two divisions of the autonomic nervous system that normally remain in balance are the sympathetic and parasympathetic systems. When this balance is severely disrupted, a state of distress is created. This results in negative effects on physical and mental functioning and behaviour. Some of the common reactions to stress are listed below.

Figure 5.1 Severity of reaction to stress is determined by a combination of environmental and individual factors

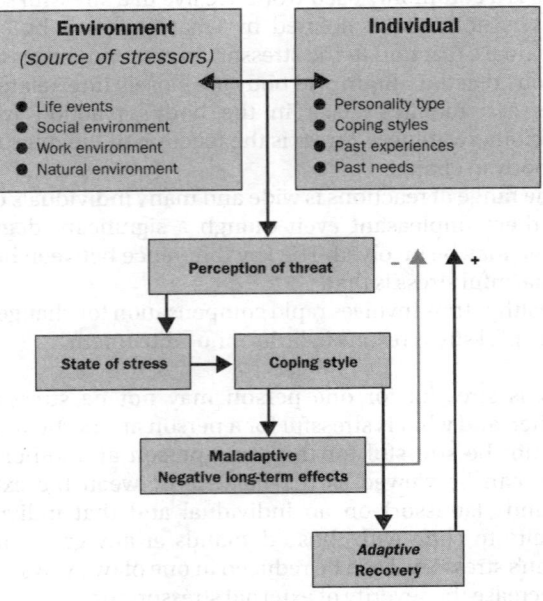

Physical effects

Physical reactions to stress manifest as:
- increased heart rate, elevated blood pressure;
- hyperventilation;
- dizziness, tingling sensations, sweating, numbness;
- muscle contractions that cause aches, pains, headaches, and tremors;
- migraine;
- gastric ulcers and nausea;
- frequent urination and diarrhoea; and
- physical illness – asthma, skin rashes, cancer.

Mental effects

The mental effects of stress manifest as:
- difficulty in concentrating;
- difficulty in making decisions;
- impaired memory – forgetfulness;
- increased negative self-critical thoughts (depressive thinking);
- distorted, irrational ideas; and
- catastrophic thinking – worrying.

Behavioural effects

The behavioural effects of stress manifest as:
- avoidance of anxiety-provoking situations;
- social withdrawal;
- excessive drinking, smoking and/or drug taking;
- disturbed sleep;
- increased aggression and/or irritation;
- accident-proneness;
- increase in obsessional tendencies;
- loss of sexual interest; and
- alteration in food intake.

Stress-related psychiatric disorders

The *Diagnostic and statistical manual of mental disorders*, 4th edn. (DSM-IV) classifies stress-induced disorders into the four categories set out below.

Adjustment disorders

Patients present with:
- adjustment disorder with depressed mood;
- adjustment disorder with anxiety;
- adjustment disorder with mixed anxiety and depressed mood;
- adjustment disorder with disturbance of conduct;
- adjustment disorder with mixed disturbance of emotions and conduct; or
- adjustment disorder with unspecified disorders.

Post-traumatic stress disorder

This disorder can be acute or chronic and can have either an early or delayed onset.

Acute stress disorder

Symptoms of post-traumatic stress disorder predominate but the condition has a short duration, namely less than one month.

Brief psychotic disorder

By definition these disorders bear a direct relationship to a significant stressor, and the severity of the symptoms depends on the severity of the stressor. It is also of less than four weeks' duration.

Psychological factors affecting a medical condition

A group of conditions presenting primarily with physical symptoms and where psychological factors are related to the onset or exacerbation of a medical disease are currently known as 'stress-related physiological response affecting a general medical condition'. In the past these conditions were referred to as psychosomatic disorders and would include illnesses such as hypertension, asthma, and irritable bowel syndrome among others.

The medical condition involves either demonstrable organic pathology or a known patho-physiological process.

Other mental disorders

There are a number of psychiatric illnesses in which stress can either precipitate an attack or may influence the progress and course of the illness. Stress factors may contribute to the onset and progress of illnesses such as schizophrenia and mood disorders.

Assessment and management

Individuals experience stress in different ways and it is therefore necessary for the PHC nurse to conduct a holistic assessment of the patient's experience. Based on this individual assessment, each patient will need an individualized plan to manage his or her stress. Table 5.1 is an example of a questionnaire that the nurse could use to assess major individual stressors.

Table 5.1 Stress assessment

Directions:
Below is a list of possible stressors taken from all aspects of life. Ask the patient to rate the items that are applicable, using the 0–4 scale.

0 = no stress
1 = little stress
2 = average
3 = very stressful
4 = extremely stressful

Table 5.1 continued

If an item is not applicable (e.g. getting married) mark with a cross on the 0. At the end of each category there is space for factors that don't appear on the list. At the end of each section, the most severe stressors from that category should be listed, before continuing to the next category.

1 Physical stressors

Excess alcohol	0	1	2	3	4
Excess substance use	0	1	2	3	4
Excess caffeine	0	1	2	3	4
Excess smoking	0	1	2	3	4
Poor eating habits	0	1	2	3	4
Poor sleeping habits	0	1	2	3	4
Regular infections	0	1	2	3	4
Poor physical shape from lack of exercise	0	1	2	3	4
Over/under weight	0	1	2	3	4
Recent surgery	0	1	2	3	4
Personal injury/illness	0	1	2	3	4
Discomfort from pain	0	1	2	3	4
Acute or chronic illness	0	1	2	3	4
Loss of sexual interest	0	1	2	3	4
Little relaxation and leisure	0	1	2	3	4
Seldom have a holiday	0	1	2	3	4
Other physical stressors					
....	0	1	2	3	4
....	0	1	2	3	4
....	0	1	2	3	4
....	0	1	2	3	4

The most important physical stressors:

1 ....

2 ....

3 ....

4 ....

2 Psychological stressors (includes emotional, intellectual, and volitional aspects)

Work is very demanding	0	1	2	3	4

Table 5.1 continued

High workload, feel overloaded	0	1	2	3	4
Unsure what is expected(poor job description)	0	1	2	3	4
Worried about relationships at the firm	0	1	2	3	4
Frustrated by relationship problems with employee/colleagues	0	1	2	3	4
Anxious due to unemployment	0	1	2	3	4
Depressed/isolated following retirement	0	1	2	3	4
Worried/anxious because recently started new job/career	0	1	2	3	4
Unwanted transfer to new department/assignment	0	1	2	3	4
Afraid, because of disciplinary steps/serious warning by boss	0	1	2	3	4
Frustrated – promotion/advancement taking longer than expected	0	1	2	3	4
Unhappy, without job satisfaction	0	1	2	3	4
Poor time management	0	1	2	3	4
Working without setting clear priorities	0	1	2	3	4
Difficulty deciding about career future	0	1	2	3	4
Not involved in decision-making	0	1	2	3	4
Can't apply effective decision-making principles (work and personal)	0	1	2	3	4
Can't delegate (want to do it myself)	0	1	2	3	4
Can't delegate (don't know the principles)	0	1	2	3	4
Blame others when things go wrong at work	0	1	2	3	4
Low motivation; boring work	0	1	2	3	4
Low motivation; poor salary	0	1	2	3	4
Little recognition; no positive feedback	0	1	2	3	4
Other psychological stressors	0	1	2	3	4
....	0	1	2	3	4
....	0	1	2	3	4
....	0	1	2	3	4
....	0	1	2	3	4

The most important psychological stressors:

1 ....
2 ....
3 ....
4 ....

Table 5.1 continued

3 Spiritual stressors (values)

Don't get on well with people, but would like to (work and personal)	0	1	2	3	4
People at work are dishonest	0	1	2	3	4
Negativity at work, no positive thinking	0	1	2	3	4
Poor communication between managers and subordinates	0	1	2	3	4
Poor communication among workers	0	1	2	3	4
Religion is negated	0	1	2	3	4
Organizational values clash with personal values	0	1	2	3	4
Can't trust anyone	0	1	2	3	4
Other spiritual stressors	0	1	2	3	4
....	0	1	2	3	4
....	0	1	2	3	4
....	0	1	2	3	4
....	0	1	2	3	4
....	0	1	2	3	4

The most important spiritual stressors:
1 ....
2 ....
3 ....
4 ....

4 Environmental stressors (work functioning, finances, political/economic influences, environment)

Irregular/long working hours	0	1	2	3	4
Boring routine, no stimulation	0	1	2	3	4
Conflict with authority/management bodies	0	1	2	3	4
Work environment without warmth/spontaneity	0	1	2	3	4
Take work home	0	1	2	3	4
Can't switch off at night – think about work	0	1	2	3	4
Don't get on with co-workers	0	1	2	3	4
Have financial problems	0	1	2	3	4
Problems paying accounts	0	1	2	3	4

Table 5.1 continued

Loss of income	....	0	1	2	3	4
Increased expenses	....	0	1	2	3	4
New bond/loan/mortgage	....	0	1	2	3	4
Large purchase/s (car, house, furniture)	....	0	1	2	3	4
Minor legal offence (e.g. traffic fine)	....	0	1	2	3	4
Prison sentence (or suspended sentence)	....	0	1	2	3	4
Unsure about the future of work in RSA	....	0	1	2	3	4
High crime and vandalism	....	0	1	2	3	4
Ethnic/racial conflict	....	0	1	2	3	4
Pollution	....	0	1	2	3	4
Noisy, unfriendly neighbours	....	0	1	2	3	4
Problems with municipal services	....	0	1	2	3	4
Problems with recreational services	....	0	1	2	3	4
Poor housing	....	0	1	2	3	4
Noise (traffic, planes, factories)	....	0	1	2	3	4
Other physical stressors						
....		0	1	2	3	4
....		0	1	2	3	4
....		0	1	2	3	4
....		0	1	2	3	4
....		0	1	2	3	4

The most important environmental stressors:

1 ....
2 ....
3 ....
4 ....

5 Social stressors (interpersonal relationships, friends, social time, support systems)

Little/no support at work	0	1	2	3	4

Table 5.1 continued

Problems with making friends	0	1	2	3	4
Deficiency of satisfying meaningful human relationships	0	1	2	3	4
Feel inferior to friends and acquaintances	0	1	2	3	4
Socially isolated	0	1	2	3	4
Feel a victim of ethnic, racial, religious, or sexual discrimination	0	1	2	3	4
Meaningful relationship ended	0	1	2	3	4
Friends live far away					
Victim of gossip and slander	0	1	2	3	4
Relationship problems with friends	0	1	2	3	4
Live alone	0	1	2	3	4
New bond/loan/mortgage	0	1	2	3	4
Other social stressors	0	1	2	3	4
....	0	1	2	3	4
....	0	1	2	3	4
....	0	1	2	3	4
....	0	1	2	3	4
....	0	1	2	3	4

The most important social stressors:

1 ....

2 ....

3 ....

4 ....

6 **Family, religion, and relationship stressors**

Ending marriage/intense love relationship	0	1	2	3	4
Marital problems	0	1	2	3	4
Divorce	0	1	2	3	4
Marital reconciliation	0	1	2	3	4
Problems disciplining children	0	1	2	3	4
Sexual problems	0	1	2	3	4
New family member	0	1	2	3	4
Poor family communication (parents/children)	0	1	2	3	4
Fights/arguments in family	0	1	2	3	4
Changed frequency in family meetings	0	1	2	3	4

Table 5.1 continued

Child with specific problems/needs	0	1	2	3	4
Severe illness in family	0	1	2	3	4
Death of spouse	0	1	2	3	4
Pregnancy of spouse	0	1	2	3	4
Not enough time for family (too busy with work)	0	1	2	3	4
Family not supportive	0	1	2	3	4
Neglect my religion	0	1	2	3	4
Seldom go to church	0	1	2	3	4
Unsure about religious commitment	0	1	2	3	4
Other spiritual stressors					
....	0	1	2	3	4
....	0	1	2	3	4
....	0	1	2	3	4
....	0	1	2	3	4
....	0	1	2	3	4

The most important relationship stressors:
1 ....
2 ....
3 ....
4 ....

7 Change stressors

Change in health of family member	0	1	2	3	4
Change to a new church	0	1	2	3	4
Change in marital status	0	1	2	3	4
Change in work hours/conditions	0	1	2	3	4
Change in residence	0	1	2	3	4
Change in living conditions	0	1	2	3	4
Other change stressors					
....	0	1	2	3	4
....	0	1	2	3	4
....	0	1	2	3	4
....	0	1	2	3	4
....	0	1	2	3	4

Table 5.1 continued

The most important change stressors:
1 ....
2 ....
3 ....
4 ....

You have now identified the most important stressors in your patient's internal and external environments, as well as the patient's patterns of interaction.

Now list the most important stressors from each category in ascending order of importance. These points may provide clues as to where you can apply stress management effectively. Keep these stressors in mind when looking at specific methods for managing stress.

This may give an indication of which area is the biggest source of stress in your patient's life. You should also fill-in a stress profile. Determine the extent to which each of the life areas contribute to your patient's stress by using the scale given at the beginning of the exercise. Using this data, create an individual stress profile (see Figure 5.2).

The stress profile as well as the individual stressors give an indication of the areas in your patient's life that require attention. The procedures described below can be used to manage stress more effectively in the life areas identified.

Elimination of stressors

The first step in managing stress is to identify any stressors that can be eliminated immediately. While it may not be possible for all stressors, some may be eliminated simply by deciding to end bad habits. For example, patients could reduce alcohol or caffeine intake, stop smoking, or plan work better. Patients can also change certain behaviour patterns or attitudes by starting, or renewing, a hobby or activity.

Figure 5.2 A stress profile

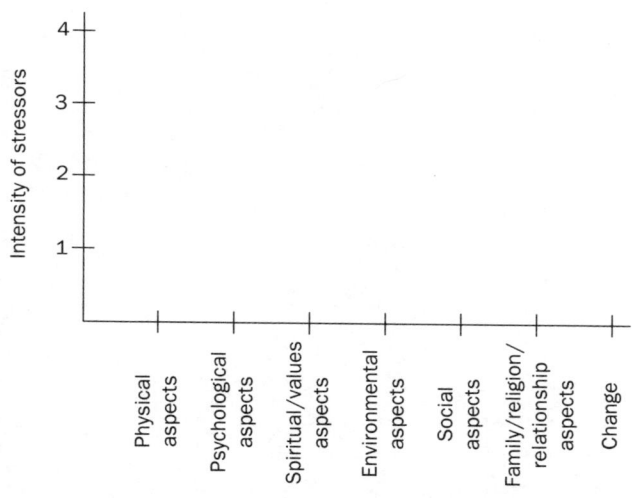

The nurse and the patient need to decide:
- which stressors the patient could change or eliminate;
- which stressors the patient could manage by changing behaviour or attitudes; and
- which activities or hobbies may have been neglected or could be undertaken.

These preliminary steps for managing stress are important and can deal with much unnecessary stress. However, patients should act on decisions taken and not simply express good intentions.

PART II
Patient care

6 Basic therapeutic competencies

Many patients suffer from chronic mental illness and have special needs that workers in the pressurized PHC situation may perceive as a nuisance. Nurses should give thought to managing these patients. For example, improved training and delegation may help nurses to improve the effectiveness of the treatment and reduce stress on staff.

Time is always limited. This chapter covers important skills that will enable the nurse to provide a good therapeutic service for mentally ill patients. Acquiring skills eventually saves time and reduces the stress on the worker. Nurses should invest in every opportunity to increase their knowledge and practise their skills under tuition.

Human relationships

A happy therapeutic team will provide the most satisfying service. Staff frictions in a clinic will have a very negative effect on patient care. One of the key functions of management is to ensure that staff maintain good working relationships with one another.

Running a service

To run an efficient service, it is important to:
- appoint a team leader based on managerial ability rather than professional or political status;
- appoint a leader who has good organizational and financial skills;
- see that staff have reasonable accommodation and working conditions, including dependable transport;
- ensure that the clinic receives regular supplies of drugs and consumables; and
- ensure that the administration is well-organized and user-friendly.

Note that a user-friendly administration is particularly important for mentally ill patients since many need understanding and especially an empathic approach.

The therapeutic team

In the smallest clinics the 'therapeutic team' will probably be one person: a doctor or a nurse. In larger clinics more people will be involved. Each individual should be regarded as having a role to play in the treatment or therapy of the patient. Apart from the more obvious members of the team, people such as cleaners, drivers, and clerks should be included in the therapeutic team and trained to maximize the full potential of their various roles in helping the patient towards health. The non-professional staff often have important contributions to make. Being heard as members of the team gives them a stake in the business of caring and healing.

Counselling skills

Nurses need to learn to listen. The basis of all effective counselling and psychotherapy is good listening. Listening requires skill and uninterrupted time even if it has to be limited. Unskilled counsellors tend to talk, interrupt too often, and give authoritative opinions on questions that the patient hasn't asked. Advice and counsel have a place only when the nurse fully understands the issues. To make the best use of even brief opportunities, all nurses need some tuition and supervision. There are many facilitative communication techniques that nurses can use to improve their counselling skills.

Techniques that facilitate effective counselling

Exploring

This is a way of gathering information on a particular subject such as the patient's feelings. For example:

Patient: 'I feel terrible today ...'
Nurse: 'Tell me what happened that made you feel so sad ...'
Nurse: 'Tell me more ...'

Reflecting (content and feelings)

Reflection entails repeating the patient's verbal or non-verbal message. Reflection conveys back to the speaker his or her:
- thoughts (reflects content); and
- feelings (reflects feelings).

Reflection of content

This is also known as validation. The nurse conveys that she or he has heard what was said and understands the content. This has a more cognitive focus, and is 'safer' for the patient. It is quite useful in the beginning of a relationship when you are getting to know one another. For example:

Patient: 'I've been wondering about working opportunities; maybe it'll be easier just to do something part-time.'
Nurse: 'You think that at this stage it will be better to take a part-time job.'

Reflection of feelings

The nurse responds to the patient's feelings about the content of the message. These responses let the patient know that the nurse is aware of what he or she is feeling. Reflection of feelings signifies understanding, empathy, interest, and respect for the patient. It is one of the most useful techniques in therapeutic communication and increases the level of trust and involvement between nurse and patient. (Beware of becoming stereotyped by beginning every reflection in the same monotonous way, such as 'you feel ... '.) For example:

Patient: 'I could kill him!'
Nurse: 'It sounds as though you're angry at your brother ...'
Patient: 'You know, I just don't know what I'll do when I leave here.'
Nurse: 'You're feeling anxious about being discharged from the hospital ...'

Imparting information

This technique is helpful in supplying the patient with additional data or factual information. Therefore further clarification is encouraged, based on new or additional input. Imparting information includes responding to direct questions with relevant facts.

Patient: 'What time is my appointment with the doctor?'
Nurse: 'Let me check in the book. Your appointment is at three o'clock.'
Patient: 'Where could I possibly go for support?'
Nurse: 'Come with me after the session and I will give you telephone numbers for various support organizations.'

Clarifying

Clarifying is an attempt to understand a patient's statement. Asking patients to give examples to clarify what they mean can help you understand the intended message better.

Patient: 'Sometimes I wonder if I really know what's going on. I feel anxious ... and sometimes not.'

Nurse: 'I'm a bit confused about this whole issue; let's go over it again.'

Clarifying what has really been said is an attempt to find the meaning of the communicated message and to establish mutual understanding.

Patient: 'Phew, that nurse … I really don't know!'
Nurse: 'I don't quite understand – what do you mean?'

Paraphrasing

The nurse assimilates and restates in similar words what the patient has said. It gives the nurse the opportunity to test his or her understanding of what a patient is attempting to communicate. It also indicates that the nurse is interested and listening.

Patient: 'My mother keeps on yelling at me as if I'm a child!'
Nurse: 'You feel like a child when your mother keeps on yelling at you.'

Checking perceptions/validating

This technique gives patients an opportunity to validate or correct your understanding of what they've said. Nurses also use perception checks to make sure they really know what their patients are communicating. They convey the message that they really care and want to understand. This technique therefore limits confusion. It is also a way to explore contradictory communication.

Nurse: 'You're smiling, but I see that you're clenching your fists … '
Nurse: 'You say you really care about her, but every time you talk about her you clench your fists. I wonder how you really feel?'
Nurse: 'It sounds as though you're very sad …'

Questioning

Every question has an intention and arises from certain assumptions. Nurses should ask questions in such a way that they create an atmosphere that facilitates dialogue, openness, sharing, and curiosity. The nurse views herself or himself as the 'non-expert' on the patient's life. This type of questioning actively draws patients into dialogue with the nurse and together they can co-construct new meanings (stories). The nurse asks questions that the patient answers. This leads to more and more questions and new meanings.

Closed-ended

Closed-ended questions limit the patient to 'yes' or 'no' answers and can also obstruct facilitative communication.

Nurse: 'Were you angry when your mother said that?'
Patient: 'Yes'

Nurse: 'Did you come here because you were forced to?'
Patient: 'No'

However, closed-ended questions are useful when communicating with patients who are experiencing high levels of anxiety or disorganized thinking. For example:

Nurse: 'Are you still hearing voices?'

Remember not to use too many closed-ended questions in succession. Too many closed-ended questions create an atmosphere of cross-examination, and the patient may become reluctant to continue. Closed-ended questions are a direct way of communicating with patients. These questions are especially useful when you need specific information, i.e., when you are assessing the patient.

Open-ended

When questioning, it is more effective to use open-ended questions than closed-ended questions. An open-ended question focuses on the topic, but allows freedom of response.

Nurse: 'How did you feel when your mother said that to you?'
Nurse: 'What do you do when … happens?'

Lineal questions: The nurse can utilize these types of questions to orientate herself or himself to the patient's 'world' based on lineal assumptions about what the patient's 'story' is. The nurse is the non-expert and conveys interest and curiosity by asking 'who', 'where', 'when', and 'why' questions. These questions stimulate answers and more questions arise. Let's look at the following example:

Nurse: 'What brought you in to see me today?'
Patient: 'I feel down and depressed.'
Nurse: 'What gets you so down?'
Patient: 'I don't know.'
Nurse: 'Who else gets depressed?'
Patient: 'My husband.'

Circular questions: These questions are mainly based on assumptions about circularity and explore circular patterns of interaction between the nurse and the patient. Circular questions, therefore, are more exploratory, i.e. the nurse discovers more about the patient's world. Remember that circular questions assume that things are connected. Everything your patients tell you is connected to many other things. These questions expose patterns that connect. Let's look at the following example:

Nurse: 'What brought you in to see me today?'
Patient: 'I feel very worried about my kids … '
Nurse: 'Who else feels worried about your kids?'
Patient: 'My husband … '
Nurse: 'Who worries the most?'
Patient: 'I do.'
Nurse: 'What do you do when you worry?'
Patient: 'I withdraw from my kids and my husband.'
Nurse: 'How do they react when you withdraw?'
Patient: 'They become angry with me and we fight.'

Strategic questions: These questions are used with a specific goal in mind. The main goal is to 'correct' behaviour that may be 'unhealthy'. These questions can be useful in challenging problematic thinking patterns and behaviour, without being too directive or dictating. Let's continue with the above example:

Nurse: 'Why don't you talk to him about these worries?'
Patient: 'He doesn't listen, he only reads the paper.'
Nurse: 'How come you're not willing to try harder to get him away from the paper to listen to you?'
Patient: 'I'm too tired to put in the effort …'
Nurse: 'Why don't you take responsibility and make the effort to get him to listen …'

This is a more direct strategy, but it can make patients look at their own world in a different way. Just be aware that this mode of inquiry may risk a disruption of the therapeutic relationship.

Reflective questions: These types of questions can influence the patient in a more indirect way, and are based on circular assumptions. They encourage patients to mobilize their own problem-solving skills. These questions also tend to open space for patients to gain new options and perspectives. For example:

Nurse: 'If you were to share with him how worried you are and how it's getting you down, what do you think he'd do?'
Patient: 'I don't know …'
Nurse: 'Let's see. If there was something he was resentful about, but didn't say so because he didn't want to hurt your feelings, how would you convince him that you could handle it?'
Patient: 'Hmm … well, tell him, I suppose!'

These questions are reflective because they help patients to reflect on the implications of their current perceptions and actions and to consider new options.

Giving feedback

It is important for patients to know or become aware of how their behaviour affects others and of how others perceive their actions. Responding with feedback can be helpful.

Therapeutic self-disclosure allows patients to become aware of their strengths and weaknesses, and to act upon them. This allows the nurse to offer patients constructive information that makes them aware of their effect on others. For instance:

Nurse: 'Sometimes when you turn your head away from me, I think you're angry.'

Confrontation

Constructive confrontation can lead to productive change. Confrontation is a deliberate invitation to examine some aspect of personal behaviour that indicates a discrepancy between what the person says and what the person does.

Confrontation is a crucial technique in facilitation, but should be used with care so that it doesn't harm your patient. Remember the following when using the confrontation technique:

- Use personal statements – 'I', 'me'.
- Use relationship statements expressing what you feel in the present.
- Confrontation must always be constructive.
- Describe the patient's behaviour; do not get personal.
- Use responses aimed at understanding, such as paraphrasing and perception checking.

Note the following example:

Nurse: 'You say you're "the black sheep" in the family, yet none of your brothers or sisters made the first team like you did.'

Focusing

This technique allows patients to deal with specifics and analyse problems without jumping from topic to topic. Focusing on feelings, thoughts, and behaviour paves the way for increased understanding, and most importantly, responsibility. Look at the following example.

Nurse: 'Rather than talking about what your husband said, I would like to hear how you are feeling about this.'

The focusing technique gets patients to concentrate on a specific thought or feeling regarding a particular point as the following example shows:

Patient: 'They are always picking on me.'
Nurse: 'I wonder who the 'they' are that you are referring to.'

Summarizing

Summarizing involves highlighting the main ideas expressed by the patient. Summarizing is useful for focusing the patient's thinking.

Nurse: 'You had three main concerns today…'
Nurse: 'The last time we were together you were most concerned about…'

The goal is to help patients to explore significant content and emotional themes. It can be used to conclude the specific interaction, or to begin a new session by reviewing a previous one.

Nurse: 'So far we've talked about…'
Nurse: 'Our time for today is up. Let's see, we've discussed your family problems, their effect on your work, and your need to find a way to decrease family conflict.'

This brings the discussion of a particular subject to a conclusion.

Silence/minimal verbal response

Silence can be of great value, but nurses often feel quite uncomfortable with this technique at first. It can be an effective facilitative technique when it encourages patients to communicate freely; when it gives them time to collect their thoughts; or when it allows them time to consider alternatives.

Silence shouldn't be uncomfortable and the nurse wouldn't want patients to become increasingly anxious and resistant. Therefore, silence is only effective when it is appropriate and purposeful. Nurses who are uncomfortable with silence or who use silence because they lack the knowledge and skills to communicate effectively must work through this before they can work actively with patients.

Minimal responses provide verbal and non-verbal reinforcement. They indicate that the nurse is listening and has an interest in what patients are saying, for example:

Nurse: 'Hmm ... hmmm ...'
Nurse: 'Yes... yes.' (Nodding head in encouragement).
Nurse: 'Go on...'
        'Uh huh...'
        'Ummm...'
Silence: Communicating without verbalization to convey interest, acceptance, and understanding.

To be able to interact with patients on a daily basis and to communicate and counsel effectively, nurses should acquire a degree of self-awareness and self-reflection. Developing self-awareness is an ongoing process. It is acquired through practice.

Non-verbal communication

Watch how patients sit, speak, and react. Observe facial expressions. This is called body language. Body language can tell you a lot about how the patient feels. A patient who doesn't maintain eye contact may be feeling ashamed, guilty, or very anxious. A patient sitting with arms and legs folded tightly may be feeling tense. If you notice this body language, then communicate, i.e. 'I see that your arms are crossed and I wonder whether you're anxious or upset?' Add to the communication by letting patients know that you're listening and in touch.

You can convey this through your own body language. Sit in a relaxed way that still indicates interest. Use phrases like 'I see and then?', 'I'm with you', 'I hear you', 'Hmm'.

7   Interviewing

Virtually all interactions in clinical psychiatry occur in the context of a consultation. This includes both diagnosis and assessment of the effect of illness on patients and their families. Since the psychiatric consultation is so important and because it works best when there is a healthy relationship between the nurse and the patient, this chapter tries to give some helpful guidelines.

Conditions during the consultation

It is important to strive for ideal conditions during consultations. Time, privacy, and consulting rooms are important factors to consider. Schedule initial consultations for approximately an hour. If you allow less time, patients will have to return for additional consultations, which heightens the risk of an incorrect diagnosis. A room that is either untidy or cramped influences the interview negatively. Patients will not be inclined to talk freely if they feel exposed. Ensure that you have privacy, quiet surroundings, and no interruptions such as telephone calls. This will contribute to an atmosphere where patients feel free to speak openly. Try to maintain eye contact, but don't force it.

Allow relatives or friends to accompany patients, if the patient desires their presence. It reduces anxiety and establishes a relationship of trust with important people in the patient's life. At some stage the patient should also be seen alone to allow for the possible sharing of information that he or she may not wish to divulge in the presence of others.

It is also important to inform the patient of the professional status of the primary care worker, i.e. whether he or she is a doctor or a nurse. The patient should be reassured that the interview is confidential.

Process and phases of the interview

The interview consists of four phases, namely:
- the relationship or orientation phase;
- the working or middle phase;
- the termination phase; and
- the feedback stage.

Relationship/orientation phase

The quality of the information revealed depends on the confidentiality and trustworthiness that the patient senses. Patients will not share personal and diagnostically important information with someone they do not trust. It is vital that patients and nurses should have good 'rapport', i.e. an understanding and trusting relationship. Elements for establishing rapport include:
- respect for patients despite their appearance or socio-economic status;
- compassion for their suffering and distress; and
- genuineness, goodwill, and an attitude that patients will find non-judgmental, interested, and concerned.

Various techniques contribute to the establishment of a sound relationship. One of the most important of these is to find, pursue, and respond to the patient's emotions and emotionally charged areas of concern. Be aware of the patient's non-verbal behaviour, listen to the suffering expressed, and respond. The ability to pick up these emotions and to respond to them with empathy conveys compassion and genuineness. Another technique that enhances rapport is to listen attentively with as little interruption as possible. Questions and probes should only be used for clarification, not for changing the direction of the interview.

Taking notes sometimes helps to avoid interrupting the patient and forms part of good record keeping. However, this must not distract the interviewer who should try to maintain eye contact throughout.

While establishing rapport, the interviewer must be aware of personal and interpersonal factors influencing the relationship, such as transference and counter-transference.

Transference: This term refers to the development of a patient's emotional attitude towards a nurse. This attitude can be either positive or negative. It includes the expectations and emotional responses that patients bring into the relationship. The patient's attitude towards the interviewer may vary from realistic trust to mistrust. When expectations are not met, patients are likely to project negative emotions and even hate. A working knowledge of the various manifestations of transference will promote the establishment of rapport.

Counter-transference: Just as the patient's transferential attitudes influence the relationship between the nurse and the patient, this relationship can also be influenced by the nurse's own counter-transferential reactions to the patient. These emotions would obviously disrupt the relationship. Patients who are compliant and grateful are usually seen positively. Patients who do not meet these expectations sometimes evoke resentment and are then seen as offensive or bad. When nurses allow themselves to dislike a patient, they disrupt good rapport. Emotion evokes counter-emotion. For instance, hostility in a nurse is likely to elicit hostility in the patient. Nurses must strive to rise above these emotions, approach the patient calmly, and replace hostility with acceptance.

Working phase/middle phase

The nurse-patient interaction enters the second step of the therapeutic relationship process when patients are able to focus on the unpleasant and often painful aspects of their lives. At this time, patients demonstrate an ability to cope with the interpersonal demands of the therapeutic process. Together, the nurse and the patient concentrate on achieving the previously identified therapeutic goals. Nursing activity is directed towards increasing the normality of the patient's behaviour. In other words, the nurse assists the patient to move toward an optimal level of functioning. The working phase is much more structured than the orientation phase. Now the nurse assists the patient to focus on ideas, themes, emotional overtones, patterns of behaviour, and coping strategies. Although structured, spontaneous interaction is encouraged, the nurse channels therapeutic communication toward the identified goals.

In the working phase the nurse has the following therapeutic tasks:

- Increase the individual's awareness and perception of the reality associated with his or her particular experiences.
- Assist the patient in developing a realistic self-concept.
- Promote the patient's self-confidence.
- Assist patients in recognizing areas of discomfort and distress by working in the present. Patients should understand the effects of their behaviour on their surroundings.
- Increase the patient's ability to describe feelings and thoughts in the present.
- Assist the patient in drawing conclusions about the effects of thoughts, feelings, and behaviour on the external environment.
- Encourage the patient to select a realistic plan of action.
- Provide opportunities for patients to implement the plan of action.
- Encourage the patient to evaluate the results of his or her behaviour.
- Provide patients with an opportunity for independent functioning and follow-up.

Termination phase

The third phase of the process is termination. The therapeutic relationship is a singularly intimate and invested encounter. The patient tends to view the therapist as a powerful force in his or her life. Therefore, nurses must be aware that when they engage in the process of termination with the patient (even if there has only been one interview), both of them need to work through and finalize this distinctly emotional and traumatic experience, which is generally referred to as separation anxiety.

Providing feedback

By the end of the interview the patient usually voices questions or concerns like: 'What is wrong with me?' or 'Will my condition improve?' Nurses should provide opportunities for patients to ask questions. They should answer fully and honestly, while avoiding technical terms and should offer appropriate reassurance. Patients must leave the interview with the impression that the nurse understands and respects them and that the information given has been conveyed to an empathic interviewer who cares, and is concerned.

8

Assessment and management of families and children

Assessment of the family

Although it is not their main focus, nurses often have to educate and manage a patient's family. Psychiatric patients usually live within a family system and these systems carry the greatest part of the burden of caring. Families act as caregivers, they support other families with similar problems, they teach and educate the patient, and they promote social re-integration and rehabilitation of the patient.

Genograms

A genogram (or family tree) is a diagrammatic, historical 'map' of three or more generations of a family. The nurse begins preparing a genogram during the first interview with the patient. Universal symbols are used to represent facts about the family. Genograms also give the patient and the family a visual image of the information that they have already given the nurse and indicate any information that is still missing. This method of gathering information enables the nurse to compose a visual image of the patient's development, genealogical relationships, and present social interaction patterns. The method also gives the patient an opportunity to expand on certain areas at a later stage.

Figure 8.1 Symbols used to denote genealogical relationships

Masculine	□	Death	✕
Feminine	○	Divorce	- - // - -
Marital relationship	—	Separation	—|—
Parent-child relationship	│	Twins (boys)	⬠⬠
Relationship	•—•	Remote relationship	•—◦
Adopted child	△	Intense relationship (over-involved)	///
Pregnancy	⊗		
Abortion	△	Relationship with conflict	∿

Figure 8.2 The family tree

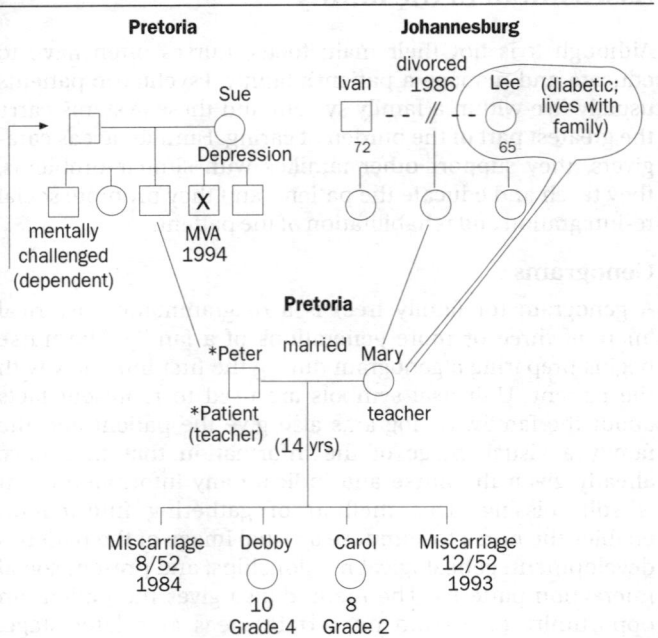

Figure 8.1 sets out some of the symbols used to represent various people and their genealogical relationships.

The nurse draws the history that the patient provides during the assessment (while taking the family history) and keeps the 'map' (visual representation) at hand to obtain more information or to work therapeutically with the patient.

Use the questions in Table 8.1 to create the genogram and to assess the patient and his or her family:

Table 8.1 Nursing assessment: genogram format

Introduce and facilitate

- List the members present for the interview and determine who initiated treatment.
- List the identified patient (IP).
- Explore the history of the presenting problem, i.e. why the family has come for help.
- Explore the history of the patient's previous hospitalization, treatments, medical and psychiatric history, and addictions.
- Explore the patient's current medical problems: whether acute or chronic, how currently managed, current medications, allergies.

Explore family history

- Ask who else in the family is symptomatic, i.e. have other family members had similar symptoms in the past?
- Explore recent life events, family transitions, and situational stressors or changes.
- Explore illnesses in the nuclear and extended family, i.e. serious medical or psychiatric illnesses or chronic pain syndrome; addictions to prescribed medications or to drugs or alcohol; violence and abuse.
- Ask about current concerns for the patient, for other family members, and for the family in general.
- Ask about the changes that the family hopes to see before ending treatment.

Formulate mutual goals and interventions

- Formulate mutual goals.
- Perform patient mental state and physical assessment.
- List family strengths and weaknesses.

Table 8.1 continued

- Record impressions and nursing diagnoses.
- Record recommendations for nursing interventions and strategies.

Explore IP's parents
(Discuss mother's family and then father's family)

- Birth order of mother/father and siblings.
- Education, occupational history, geographic locations over time, health history.
- Birth and death dates; From what did each die?
- What does the IP remember about his or her mother's/father's family and specifically about his or her mother/father?
- What does he or she remember most about his or her mother/father?
- What was the mother/father like?
- What traits of theirs does the IP have?
- What traits has the IP passed on to the children?
- Ask the IP to share an important moment between him or herself and his or her mother/father?
- To which parent did he or she feel closer; Why?
- Was there any distance or conflict between the IP and one parent (ask reason)?
- Are any family members in the extended family especially close?
- Do any family members not speak to each other (or have they ever had a period of not speaking to each other? Are there issues of conflict)?
- Explore problem(s): How have relationships been influenced by the issue or problem?
- What does the future hold for the family?
- What will happen in the family if the problem continues or if it goes away?

Discuss IP's courtship and marriage(s)

- Ask what each partner was doing when they met.
- What attracted them to each other?
- Explore where each was born and educated, and their work history.
- Ask whether either partner had any physical, emotional, or social symptoms prior to their meeting or during their courtship, early marriage, etc.
- How/where/when did the spouse(s) meet?

Table 8.1 continued

- Ask what else was happening in the family when they were contemplating marriage.
- Ask about the wedding, i.e. who came, who didn't and the reasons; Who was not invited (ask why)?
- What kinds of things did they enjoy doing together as a young couple?
- Explore earlier marriages and divorces and issues of conflict.
- Where are ex-spouse(s) and children by that marriage now? What is the current relationship? What are their occupations?
- Determine who has lived with the couple over time.
- What does the couple disagree about?
- What sorts of conflicts and problems have they had (or do they currently have)?
- Explore the birth order of the spouses and relevant family members; Determine issues and patterns.

Discuss IP's child(ren)
(This relates to children conceived inside or outside of the couple's marriage[s])

- How did the IP/the spouse/family react to the pregnancies/birth(s) of the children?
- Was anyone in the family sick during any pregnancy or in the early months after any birth?
- How does/did the IP get along with each of the children?
- Who is/was closest to whom?
- What kinds of things did the couple enjoy doing with their children when they were growing up?
- What were the most pleasurable ages or stages of development?
- Did any of the children have problems as young children, teenagers, or young adults?
- Do any of the children have any difficulties now?
- Have any recent job changes, unemployment, or work changes occurred?
- Which child(ren) have gotten married, separated, or divorced?
- Which child(ren) have children? How many? How old? Are any of them in college, service, or careers?
- Do any problems exist between any of the children or grand-children?
- Do any of the family members frequently take prescribed medications?

Table 8.1 continued

- Do any of the children or grandchildren have problems with drugs or alcohol?
- Has anyone in the family been ill, moved away, had an accident, died, or been arrested?
- What do they think the future holds for the family and for particular family members?

Family support – nursing interventions

Getting to know the family

This has to do with the approach that nurses use when they introduce themselves to and greet a family. It involves building rapport (a sense of connection) from early on by showing support and caring. This takes place during the orientation or relationship phase of family counselling.

Problem solving

Problem solving (also called psychoeducation) involves taking a systematic approach to problems. This is a useful technique for any family to learn. Work through the following steps with the family:

- *Define the problem:* 'We need to talk about why you have all come here today. I would like to hear from everyone.'
- *Explore solutions:* Encourage each member of the family to offer solutions, without allowing the other members to judge them. The suggestions can be jotted down and evaluated on a form such as the one in Table 8.2.
- *Choose a solution:* The family agrees on the solution that has the most positive and the least negative implications.
- *Implement the solution:* The family agrees on what has to be done, by when, and by whom.
- *Give feedback:* Once the family members have implemented their plans, encourage them to arrange another appointment for feedback. Here you can evaluate the family's progress in addressing the problems and assess whether ongoing work is necessary.

Table 8.2 Form for evaluating solutions to problems

Solutions (All possible solutions)	Positive points (Positive aspects of the suggestion)	Negative points (Negative aspects of the suggestion)
Solution 1		
Solution 2		
Solution 3		

Structuring the session

Although it is useful to set appointments, practical problems may make it difficult for the family to return for further consultation. For this reason, each session should constitute a complete intervention so that the family leaves with the appropriate tools (skills that they have learnt from the nurse during the session) to manage their problem. Alternatively, they must be referred elsewhere to continue working on the problem. Sometimes, they will require only one counselling session and one feedback session.

Referral

Although the need for specialist referral is discussed in Chapter 1, primary care is provided in a community setting and there are possibilities for referral within the community. When nurses encounter specialized problems such as substance abuse or juvenile delinquency, they may need to refer these patients to other agencies. Similarly, families that need ongoing support should be encouraged to contact and use the resources within their own communities. Nurses cannot be expected to take full responsibility in this regard, but they can feel free to provide the names of contacts.

Referral is indicated in cases of:

- persistent symptoms of adjustment problems;
- the existence of mood-, post-traumatic-, and anxiety disorders;

Table 8.3 An example of listed community resources

Organization	Telephone number	Address	Contact person	Services offered
FAMSA				
Psychiatric community services				
Churches				
Traditional healers				
Local civics				

- the involvement of a child;
- the occurrence of multiple deaths; and/or
- one family member having been involved in the death of another.

Nurses would be well advised to list the appropriate resources in the community and to distribute these lists among colleagues who may add to them (see Table 8.3).

Assessment of children

The child psychiatric interview is intended as a guide to interviewing children. It is not a checklist, nor is it intended to be all-inclusive. Where specific information is required, for example with abused, depressed, psychotic, or autistic children, refer patients for more specialized interviews.

After thorough assessment of a child, the nurse formulates a preliminary diagnosis and manages the child accordingly, or refers the child for more specialized treatment. It is usually appropriate to refer all cases of sexual abuse to a specialist child abuse clinic for more intensive individual or group

Table 8.4 Child psychiatric interview

Introduction and interviewing

- Escort the child to and from the waiting room.
- Welcome the child and set her or him at ease.
- Use play and observation with younger children initially, then move into verbal communication.
- Reassure children that their confidence will not be betrayed unless the information has to be revealed in a report for court (in which case an explanation to the child is necessary).
- Discuss the reason for referral, i.e. 'What do you call this place?' 'Do you know why children come here?'.
- Arrange to have useful materials such as drawing materials, construction toys (e.g. Lego, blocks), and a family of dolls.

As far as possible, the rest of the room should be free of toys or other distracting objects.

General questions

These include general topics and conversation about recent events and activities.

- What does he or she like doing on weekends?
- What television does he or she watch?
- What are his or her hobbies or interests, and what games are played?
- What would he or she like to be when grown up (ambitions and aspirations)?
- Ask the child to make three wishes.
- Ask the child to imagine being alone on an island – who would he or she take as a companion and why?
- Ask the child to draw whatever he or she likes and to tell a story about the drawing on completion, i.e. free drawing.

Structure and specific questions

- *School:* How are you doing at school? Do you have homework? Who helps you? What do you like best and least? Why? Do you like or dislike the teacher? Why? Do you like or dislike your subjects? Why? What activities do you like or dislike? Why?
- *Peers:* Do you have one special friend? Enquire about teasing, bullying, or anxieties. Specify peer contacts and determine if the child is popular or isolated. Do you ever feel lonely?

Table 8.4 continued

- *Appetite:* Do you like eating? Enquire about eating patterns. Enquire about weight loss or gain.
- *Sleep:* Do you like or dislike getting up in the morning? What about going to sleep at night? Enquire about sleep problems.
- *Dreams:* What do you dream about? Do you have bad, nasty, or scary dreams? How often? Do you wake up? Who comforts you?
- *Worries:* Explain that many people worry. What kinds of things do you worry about? Does thinking about unpleasant or nasty things ever stop you from getting to sleep? Do you ever get nasty, unhappy, or worrying thoughts? What is your biggest worry?
- *Depression:* Do you ever cry? Do you feel really unhappy some-times? Do you sometimes feel sad for no reason?
- *Fears:* Many children are afraid of things like snakes or spiders. Enquire about fears of shadows, dark, ghosts, cats, dogs, etc. Are these fears in the past or present? What do you do when you meet whatever things you are afraid of? Are you afraid of things happening to you or your family? What kind of things?
- *Anger:* Everyone gets angry sometimes – what makes you angry? What do you do when you are angry? Do you get into fights some-times? Do you like fighting? Are they 'friendly' or 'real' fights? Who do you fight with? How often? What makes you stop being angry?
- *Home:* Who lives there? What is father/mother's work? Do you have your own bedroom? Who do you get on best with? Do you have any brothers or sisters? We all have fights with siblings – do you fight often? Are they real or friendly fights?

therapy and medico-legal assistance. The primary care work-er's involvement and support is an important aspect of this work.

Understanding children's behaviour

When working with parents and children, some of the princi-ples of STEP (discussed below) can be very useful. They can aid in understanding certain behaviours in children, and assist in conveying these insights to parents. STEP stands for Systematic Training for Effective Parenting and provides a framework for parents to understand and manage their children effectively. This helps them to build and maintain healthy relationships and encourages children to grow into healthy adults who take responsibility for their own actions, feelings, and thoughts.

All young children have power struggles with parents and parents often express an inability to deal with these behaviours. They worry that if they 'punish' children, they could psychologically scar them, but that if they leave them to do as they please, children may not grow into responsible adults.

Parents often also wonder why their children misbehave. There is usually a reason for particular behaviour. Children need to feel that they belong and are accepted. To do this, they will behave or misbehave. Understanding how children try to belong is important in helping parents to become more effective. Psychologist Rudolf Dreikurs (Dinkmeyer, McKay and Dinkmeyer, 1997) discovered that when children misbehave, they are *discouraged*. They want to belong, but they do not believe they can belong in useful ways. They find that misbehaviour pays off. Dreikurs identified four main goals of misbehaviour. Knowing these goals can help the nurse to understand misbehaviour and guide children towards more positive behaviour.

The four goals of misbehaviour

When children misbehave they have a goal. They may feel the only way to belong is by:
- attention;
- power;
- revenge; or
- displays of inadequacy.

Attention
All children need attention, but some children seem to want attention all the time. When they can't get attention in useful ways, they get it by misbehaving. For example, they will do something to annoy their parents. When parents step in to correct the misbehaviour, the child has thier attention. However, it's not long before the child wants more attention.

Sometimes children ask for attention more quietly. A child might do nothing, expecting to be waited on, which is called passive misbehavior. It is still a bid for attention.

Power

Some children believe they can belong only by being the 'boss'. Their goal is power. A child who seeks power is telling the parent, 'I am in control', 'You can't make me!' or 'You'd better do what I want!'. The child might yell these things or fight out loud with the parent. Or the child might silently refuse to budge.

When a child seeks power, the parent feels angry. If the parent fights the child, the child fights back. If the parent gives in, the child has won the power struggle and so stops misbehaving.

Sometimes a child will do what the parent wants, but will do it extremely slowly or sloppily. This is a form of passive power. The child is saying, without words, 'All right, I'll do it – just to get you off my back. But I'll do it my way. You can't make me do it your way.'

Revenge

Some children want to be in charge but can't win in a power struggle with their parents. These children decide that the way to belong is to get even. Dreikurs called this goal revenge. A child who wants revenge may say or do something hurtful. Or the child may stare angrily at the parent. Either way, the parent feels hurt and angry and tries to get even. The result is often a growing 'war' of revenge. Both the child and the parent are hurt and angry.

Displaying inadequacy

Some children just give up. For them, the way to belong is to get others to leave them alone. Their behaviour says, 'I can't do it'. Dreikurs called this displaying inadequacy. When a child gives up, the parent feels like giving up too. When this happens, the child's goal has been met. The parent has agreed to expect nothing from the child.

For most children, this helplessness is not total. It usually happens in certain areas of the child's life. This might be in schoolwork, sports, or other social activities. It can be in any area where the child feels unable to succeed.

Children don't know that their misbehaviour has a goal. Children may also use the same behaviour to achieve different goals. Be aware that parents don't cause children's misbehavior. By their own behaviour though, they may reinforce it. The key to assessing the goal of a child's misbehaviour is to look at the three clues: how the parent feels, what the parent does, and how the child responds.

9

History taking the and mental state examination (MSE)

In a primary health care clinic, patients often present with physical complaints not related to a medical condition. Therefore, the initial assessment will be as for any other patients who present at the primary health care clinic.

A holistic assessment must be done and therefore it is necessary to:

- take a *clear history* of the complaints;
- perform a thorough *physical examination*;
- concentrate on certain areas in the history if you suspect a psychiatric disorder; and
- examine the person's *mental state* as part of the central nervous system (CNS) examination.

While the patient is being interviewed the history-taker observes the psychiatric symptoms and signs the patient is presenting with. This is called the *mental state examination* and will be discussed later in this chapter. (Note that the history gives the nurse a long-term view of the patient while the mental state examination gives her or him a view of the patient's status at the time of the exam.)

Before the nurse examines the patient's mental state, she or he will do a physical examination. Use the guidelines that follow.

General physical and medical examination

It is essential to do a thorough physical examination on every patient who presents with a psychiatric symptom. This is *especially important* if the patient is confused, because many physical diseases, both inside the brain, and in the rest of the body may present with psychiatric symptoms. If the correct diagnosis is not made, and correct treatment started soon, this can be very dangerous. The nurse should:

- Check the patient's vital signs (temperature, pulse, blood pressure, breathing).
- Check the skin, colour, and lesions. This might suggest anaemia, Aids, alcoholism, syphilis.
- Test the patient's urine (glucose, protein, blood, bilirubin).
- Check the nutritional status and weight of the patient (TB, pellagra, malnutrition, alcoholism).
- Check for enlargement of the thyroid gland.

Other special investigations

Other special investigations that may be required are:

- a full blood count (FBC);
- a liver function test (LFT);
- a white cell count;
- a lithium level test (if the patient is on lithium);
- a thyroid function test (if it appears to be enlarged or if the patient has symptoms suggestive of thyroid disease); and
- an EEG and skull X-ray and/or CT scan (if indicated) when organic brain pathology is expected.

Psychiatric history taking

General points

- Build a trusting relationship with the patient, express warmth and empathy, and explain every action.
- Allow the patient to explain the problem initially in his or her own words, and spend some time getting to understand the exact nature of the patient's problem.

Be especially careful if there is a language difficulty. If necessary, use a translator.

- Avoid leading questions, for instance, 'You do have headaches, don't you?' or 'Do you have headaches?' These are threatening. Ask open-ended questions: 'Tell me about …' or 'Tell me more …'
- A framework for a mental state examination is useful when conducting an assessment interview in order not to miss essential information (see p.113).
- Write down exactly what the patient says (in his or her own words) especially if it sounds strange or different from normal. Quote the patient's own words.

Structured history-taking method

(See the summary in Table 9.1 on pp. 104 to 106.)

Demographic data

The patient is a 29-year-old white male who has never been married, has no children, lives alone, has to be cared for in a 'halfway house', and is unemployed. He passed matric, and is a non-practising Methodist.

Comment

This information tells us that, despite a reasonable level of education, this patient is not functioning and needs semi-structured care. Demographic data tells us about the patient's socio-cultural background and helps us to understand him in his context.

Main complaint

His main complaint is that voices speak to him and tell him that people are planning to destroy him by reading his innermost thoughts. He firmly believes that these voices are real and that the threat to him is real. As a result he is distressed, not eating well, and having difficulty in sleeping soundly. He is unable to work and shuts himself in his room all day. No amount of coaxing or explaining can change his convictions. According to his family, he is 'mad'.

Comment

The patient is probably psychotic and the psychosis is imped-
ing his ability to function.

History of present illness

The present episode began three months ago. He first started
hearing sounds and felt that people were looking at him in a
strange way. Within a matter of two weeks these symptoms
had progressed. At first the patient tried to hide the symptoms from others, because this would mean that he would
have to restart medication and risked being hospitalized
again. He had not taken any medication for the month prior
to the onset of the symptoms. No other major changes had
occurred in his life during the last three years.

Comment

The relapse was probably a result of having discontinued
medication. Relapse was not sudden but set in over a period
of weeks.

There were no other significant stressors. The patient
was reluctant to report for treatment. In a case like this
one, the nurse should remain empathetic and not give any
indication of possible exasperation at his poor compliance.
This would merely serve to make him even less co-operative.

Past psychiatric history

The patient first began hearing voices when he was eighteen
years old and in matric. Although he passed, he did not do as
well as expected. In his first year at university the voices and
paranoid beliefs became so intense that he had to give up his
studies and was hospitalized for the first time. Since then he has
been admitted to psychiatric wards or hospitals on six occasions. On each of these occasions, antipsychotic medication has
been prescribed and this has relieved the symptoms. However,
he has not been able to resume his studies. In his early twenties
he was able to work in a grocery store. For the last four years he
has been unemployed. Each time he has relapsed it has been
because he has stopped taking his medication. His reason for

stopping has been his insistence that he is not ill and that he was unable to tolerate the side-effects of the medication.

Comment

Since the onset of the illness, the patient's level of functioning has steadily declined.

Despite the effectiveness of the medication in controlling symptoms he lacks insight. Side-effects to medication are a problem.

Systematic inquiry of psychiatric symptoms

The symptoms not already investigated under the above headings should now be followed up.

The patient admits that he is very depressed, cannot stand the tension the voices are provoking in him, and just wishes he was dead. Despite this he has no active plans to kill himself. He has no history of ictal symptoms (epilepsy). At times he becomes extremely anxious and experiences full-blown panic attacks. He has no other anxiety features, nor is there evidence of any eating disorder.

Comment

Other psychiatric symptoms such as mood and anxiety features tend to arise as a result of the psychotic phenomena. This systematic inquiry ensures that other significant symptoms are not missed.

Family psychiatric history

His father committed suicide when the patient was eleven years old. He knows nothing about him except that he spent many years in various psychiatric hospitals. His mother is diabetic and lives on her own. He has no siblings, and did not know his grandparents.

Comment

Many psychiatric illnesses have a genetic component. The father suffered from a serious psychiatric condition. This was not a close family and there is little information.

Given the mother's diabetes, the patient's glucose must be checked. Diabetes may affect both his psychiatric symptoms and their treatment.

Present medical/surgical status

The patient is not on any other medication, and has no symptoms indicating a physical disability.

Comment

The presence of any co-existing medical illness, besides being a possible cause of the psychiatric presentation, should make the nurse especially careful in managing the patient and should serve as a warning to be on the look-out for possible drug interaction.

Previous medical/surgical history

The patient has had no previous operations, head injuries, or serious physical problems in the past.

Comment

Physically, at least, he has always been healthy.

Allergies

No known allergies.

Comment

Find out whether the patient is allergic to specific medications so that these can be avoided.

Habits

The patient admits to smoking cannabis about twice a week. He takes no alcohol, but smokes up to forty cigarettes and drinks the equivalent of ten cups of coffee a day. He denies taking any over-the-counter (OTC) medications.

Comment

The use of psychoactive substances is very common among psychiatric patients. Try to understand why the patient takes substances – probably to escape from the harshness of the illness. Street drugs and socially acceptable psychoactive substances do nevertheless influence the clinical picture. Caffeine may aggravate his underlying anxiety and be the trigger that provokes his panic attacks.

Personal history

This patient was born by Caesarian section after a prolonged labour. His mother described him as a rather clingy and shy child. She ascribed this to the fact that she had never married his father, and that the patient had never had any contact with his father, who did not live with them. At school he was a loner who passed each standard but did not excel in sport. He did not do as well as expected in matric, and could not cope with university. His subsequent employment record was erratic and he had no job stability. Socially he became even more withdrawn and spent most of his time alone. Throughout his life he made no friends. His only sexual encounters had been heterosexual and fleeting. He spent most of his time sitting in his room smoking.

Comment

This helps us establish an understanding of the patient and his life. It is useful to plot a rough graph that then gives us a pattern and an overall impression (Figure 9.1).

Figure 9.1 Function/treatment graph

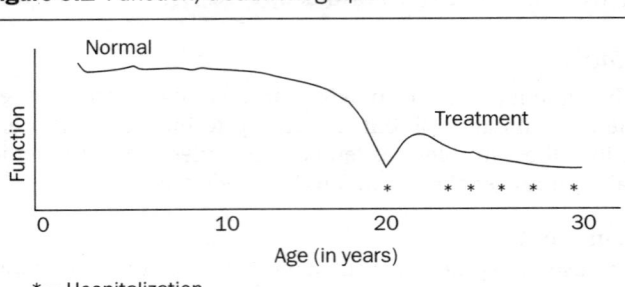

* = Hospitalization

In this patient, for instance, early development and schooling was relatively normal. A gradual decline preceded a psychotic breakdown. Since the breakdown there have been few signs of recovery.

Personality assessment

The patient's mother described him as a lonely, shy person who did not take responsibility for himself and tended to live in a world of his own. He did not allow people to get either physically or emotionally close to him. The patient was unable to describe himself in any detail.

Comment

This shows the importance of collateral information. His mother describes someone with schizoid and avoidant traits.

Present circumstances

As already mentioned, this patient is unemployed and stays in a halfway house. He is not in trouble with the law and has no close family ties.

Comment

Understand the patient in context: what kind of person has the disorder?

Summary: main points from the history

A 29-year-old unemployed male has a three-month history of worsening psychosis after having discontinued medication. There were six previous episodes of psychosis with admissions. The previous diagnosis was schizophrenia. Haloperidol and trifluoperazine were administered with good response but bad side-effects. The overall function between relapses was poor and was worsening. The patient uses cannabis, caffeine, and OTC (over-the-counter) medication, but denies it.

There is a positive family history of suicide and diabetes. The patient has schizoid and avoidant personality traits, but no history of any medical illness of note.

Table 9.1 History taking: summary

1 **Demographic data**
   ● Name
   ● Age
   ● Marital status
   ● Children
   ● Accommodation
   ● Employment
   ● Education
   ● Religion

2 **Main complaint**
   ● Get as much detail as necessary.
   ● Determine the impact on appetite, weight, sleep, sex, energy (these are the vegetative symptoms).
   ● Determine the impact on social, occupational, and leisure functioning.

3 **History of present illness**
   ● Search for an underlying cause.
   ● Determine the acuteness of onset (whether gradual or rapid).
   ● Determine the progression over time.
   ● Determine the precipitating, perpetuating, predisposing, and relieving factors.
   ● Find out whether there are secondary problems such as clashes with the law.

4 **Past psychiatric history**
   ● Establish the pattern of psychiatric presentations and their effect on the patient's life.
   ● Note the level of functioning between episodes of the illness and how well the patient responded to previous methods of treatment.

5 **Systematic inquiry of psychiatric systems**
   ● Mood symptoms: neurovegetative symptoms, cognitive features, both high and low moods, suicidal tendencies.
   ● Psychotic symptoms: delusions, hallucinations, illusions, racing thoughts, slow thoughts, lost thoughts, other people reading thoughts.
   ● Ictal symptoms (epilepsy): episodic mood changes, perceptual disturbance (all sensory modalities), memory disturbances

Table 9.1 continued

(deja vu, jamais vu, premonitions), dissociative states (depersonalization, fugue states). All of the above may occur before, during, or after seizure.

6 Family psychiatric and medical history
- Psychiatric illnesses and response to treatment
- Alcohol or drug problems
- Suicide
- Neurological or medical conditions

7 Present medical or surgical status (including present medications)
- Systematic questioning

8 Previous medical or surgical status
- Relevant previous investigations and responses to treatment
- Head injuries
- Loss of consciousness

9 Allergies
- Check to avoid undesirable medication.

10 Habits
- Include caffeine and over-the-counter (OTC) medications.

11 Personal history
The personal history is usually divided into the major developmental periods, namely prenatal and infancy, childhood, adolescence, and adulthood.
Prenatal and infancy
- Mother's pregnancy and delivery, prematurity, planned pregnancy
- Temperament and behavioural problems
- Milestones

Childhood
- School adjustment, relationships with peers and teachers
- Hyperactivity or learning difficulties
- Presence of nightmares, phobias, bedwetting, masturbation, and antisocial behaviour or criminal activities
- Who was the main caregiver, where, for what period?

Table 9.1 continued

> *Adolescence*
> - Emotional or physical problems, and psychosexual development
>
> *Adulthood*
> - Advanced education and occupation(s)
> - Social activities
> - Marital history
> - Adult sexuality
> - Employment history
> - Contact with noxious substances, e.g. heavy metals

12 Personality assessment
- Lifelong and habitual attitudes and patterns of behaviour (may be affected by the illness)
- Locus of control, i.e. blames other people and events or takes personal responsibility
- Establish into which personality cluster the patient best fits (see Chapter 17).

Note: a full personality assessment is only possible with the aid of collateral information.

13 Present life circumstances
- Income
- Relationships

The mental state examination (MSE)

See the summaries of the mental state examination (MSE) on p. 113 and of the mini-mental state examination (MMSE) on p. 212 of Chapter 19.

Overview

The patient is thin, prematurely balding but with long scraggly hair. He is casually dressed in jeans and a T-shirt. He is unshaven and does not appear to have washed for a few days. He is barefoot.

The patient makes little attempt at contact and answers questions as briefly as possible, answering some reluctantly and refusing to elaborate on others. At times he is clearly bored, and at others is not paying attention to the interviewer. At times it looks as though he is listening to someone else speaking.

He has continual lip and tongue movements, as if he is chewing gum, although he has nothing in his mouth. He is rather fidgety and has difficulty sitting still.

Despite his reluctance to co-operate, the patient does not appear to be lying at any time during the interview. He does appear to be concerned about happenings of which we may not be aware.

Comment

This initial overview is one of the most significant parts of the MSE. It helps the clinician to assess what sort of contact there is with the patient. If the patient is uncooperative (as in this case) it is necessary to establish why. Is he deliberately trying to mislead the clinician or is he so preoccupied by his illness and symptoms that he cannot focus on the questions or even acknowledge the clinician's presence? Is something interfering with his thought processes?

The patient is poorly groomed, makes poor contact, is uncooperative and shows evidence of tardive dyskinesia. Although he is not deliberately trying to mislead the clinician, he is too preoccupied by his illness to be assessed as being 'reliable'.

Sensorium

The patient is orientated in terms of person, time, and place. He is awake and shows a clear conscious state. He does, however, show considerable distractability and will not even attempt to do formal tests of concentration (serial 7s or serial 3s).

Comment

Only if the patient has a clear sensorium, will the rest of the MSE be valid. A confused and drowsy patient is more often than not suffering from either a medical or toxic condition. Poor concentration on its own may be due to both medical and psychiatric disorders. This particular patient is too distracted by his own psychosis to be able to concentrate or co-operate.

Memory

The patient is able to recall six digits forward and four backward. He remembers four objects after five and ten minutes, but does require prompting. When pressed, he is able to give an accurate account of significant dates and events in his life.

Comment

When this patient is able to concentrate, his memory is intact. From assessing how well and accurately the patient answers questions during the history taking, an initial impression of his memory function may be gleaned before proceeding to the more formal tests.

Speech and language

The patient speaks in a monotone. He has a very soft voice with few inflections. At times he slurs his speech and hesitates. There are often long pauses between sentences.

Comment

This picture shows both a lack of concentration and some minor problems with articulation. The long-term effects of medication may well play some role in this patient's speech difficulties.

Cognitive functions

When asked to draw a bicycle, the patient draws two circles connected by a straight line with no further detail. He is able to do simple calculations involving addition and subtraction, but has difficulty with anything more complex. When asked about the similarity between an apple and an orange he replies that they are both round. He is unable to say why a banana and an apple are similar. Throughout the interview, the patient remains suspicious of the clinician. When asked why, he eventually answers that, as the clinician is able to read his thoughts anyway, he sees no point in talking too much. He will often light a cigarette without requesting permission. At one stage during the interview he picks his nose and passes wind.

Comment

The cognitive functions are tested in order to assess the patient's present level of intellectual functioning. This provides an overall impression of his intelligence, highlights certain areas of possible deficits, and will give an indication of gross problem areas. In order to define deficits more accurately, sophisticated neuropsychological tests may have to be done by a psychologist.

It is obvious that this patient pays very little attention to detail. He shows a deficiency in concrete reasoning in that he is unable to conceptualize the various objects as 'fruit'. His social judgement is lacking in that he is unaware that some of his actions may be offensive to the interviewer. Overall his intelligence does not appear to be on the level of someone who has passed matric.

Note that the above conclusions are only valid for a patient who has had at least five years of formal education. Questions for a patient who is illiterate or innumerate, will have to be tailored to his or her level of sophistication and socio-cultural background. Using proverbs will test learned rather than deductive intelligence.

Mood and emotions

The patient admits to feeling tense and depressed (mood). Objectively he certainly appears tense and is withdrawn (affect). At times his behaviour is inappropriate, given the content of the interview in that he is unduly frightened by apparently routine questions. He does not show much mood lability and appears to show little depth of emotion. He is 'blunted' in that he shows little facial expression or change in voice modulation. When discussing potentially emotive topics, he shows very little concern for or awareness of the seriousness of the topic at hand.

Comment

The purpose here is to assess the patient's emotional depth and appropriateness as well as his present mood state. This patient, while showing signs of depression, is very superficial and often acts inappropriately. He is, however, generally in control of his emotions. There are no anger outbursts nor is there excessive tearfulness. He is neither aggressive nor grandiose.

Thoughts

The patient speaks slowly with many pauses. At times his answers are disjointed and do not quite make sense. The content is clearly delusional. He also talks about having an 'orthodromic heart condition'.

Comment

The speed with which the patient speaks gives us some indication of his efficiency in processing his thoughts. Speed may be slowed as in psychomotor retardation or speeded up as in pressure of thought and flight of ideas.

Form of thought gives an indication of the logic the patient is using. Thought form is often difficult to describe. Various kinds of thought form should be looked for: normal thought, circumstantial thought (many inclusions before reaching the point), tangential thought (never gets to the point), loosening of association, incoherence, or loss of association.

A disturbance in the form or organization of the patient's thoughts is often referred to as 'formal thought disorder'. This differentiates it from a disorder of thought content.

The patient shows evidence of a disorder of both form and content of thought. He has psychomotor retardation and loosening of association (form). He is clearly paranoid to the point of being delusional (content). His use of the word 'orthodromic' is a good example of a neologism, which is a word that does not appear in any dictionary (a made up word).

Note: neologisms are easily missed in translation and the translator should be specifically asked to look out for them.

Perceptual disturbances

In the history this patient admits to hearing voices and appears to be listening to someone else speaking.

Comment

This patient is subjectively and objectively hallucinating.

Insight

The patient does not question the reality of his beliefs or hallucinations.

Comment

This patient has no insight into the fact that he is experiencing false beliefs (delusions) or perceptual disturbances in the absence of an outside stimulus (hallucinations). In other words he is psychotic. This lack of insight is the hallmark of a psychosis.

- *Full insight* describes patients who know that they are ill and understand the illness and its implications for their lives.
- *Partial insight* occurs when patients are aware that there is an illness present, but are not fully aware of the impact or finer points of the condition.
- *No insight* implies the denial of even the possibility of being ill.

The patient being dealt with here has neither insight into the fact that he is ill, nor into the implications of the illness on his life.

General comments

The MSE starts from the time the patient is first seen and continues throughout the interview. Indeed, formal questioning is only a minimal part of the MSE.

All the MSE does is give us an indication of how the patient is at this present moment, i.e. a cross-sectional view. The history gives a longitudinal view.

The symptoms and signs derived from the MSE are subsequently combined with the information derived during history taking.

Summary: main points from MSE

The patient was unkempt and clearly psychotic. He showed evidence of poor social judgement, delusions, hallucinations, and a formal thought disorder. His emotions were superficial and he was depressed and expressed a wish to die.

Physical examination revealed a thin young man with evidence of tardive dyskinesia. No other abnormalities were detected.

From the preceding history, MSE, and summary, it is clear that this patient is suffering from a chronic remitting and relapsing psychotic condition.

The next step is to decide what psychiatric syndrome most closely fits this picture, to proceed with appropriate special investigations (medical or psychological) and, wherever possible, obtain a detailed collateral history.

Formulation/diagnosis

The main features of the history, MSE, physical and special investigations, and collateral history, can be summarized in what is called a 'formulation'. The DSM-IV format for this patient would be as follows (see Appendix 2, p. 329):

Axis I   –   Psychiatric diagnosis: schizophrenia.

Axis II   –   Personality and development: schizoid and avoidant traits (premorbid), normal development (premorbid).

Axis III –   Medical illness: nil.

Axis IV   –   Psychosocial stressors: nil at present.

Axis V   –   Assessment of function (occupation, social interaction, use of leisure): low since first episode (function between episodes low even when psychosis is controlled).

Nursing diagnosis

Bizarre behaviour and thought disturbance related to inability to cope with pressures of daily living, secondary to family history of psychiatric illness, as evidenced by:

- isolation;
- auditory hallucinations;
- paranoid ideation/delusions;

- distractibility/poor concentration;
- problems with articulation;
- deficiency in concrete reasoning;
- social judgement lacking;
- blunted affect;
- thought disturbance (form and content);
- neologisms; and
- lack of insight.

Table 9.2 summarizes the mental state examination.

Table 9.2 Mental state examination (MSE): summary

Overview
General appearance (e.g. description of person, grooming, etc.), contact, co-operation, motor behaviour, reliability

Sensorium
- Orientation
- Conscious state
  - clear/clouded/drowsy/awake/aware
- Concentration
  - e.g. serial 7s, months backwards

Memory
Three phases of memory: recording, retaining, and recalling (memory can only be tested accurately if concentration is intact).

Memory test
- Immediate recall (six digits forward/four digits backward)
- Short-term (give four objects to remember – house, tree, cloud, flight; ask again in 5 minutes)
- Long-term (dates and events)

Note: Modify expectations to accommodate education and culture.

Speech and language
Assess mechanics of speech, including tone, volume, and pronunciation, grammatical construction, and form. Look for features of dysphasia – if present, try to assess type of dysphasia.

Note: Translator needs training to pick this up.

Table 9.2 continued

Cognitive functions

This is aimed at a global assessment of the patient's cognitive capacities and comparing this with what you would expect from the patient in a healthy state. Consider education, culture, and language.

Functions to be tested

- Constructional ability (e.g. draw a bicycle)
- Calculations
- Capacity to think in abstract terms (similarity between banana and orange)
- Judgement and planning ability (observe the patient's social judgement – real-life examples)
- Clinical assessment of intelligence: vocabulary, calculations, general knowledge, etc.

Mood and emotions

Assess how the patient feels (mood) and how the patient appears (affect) and anxiety features; neurovegetative features are elicited during the history.

- Observe for:
  - appropriateness/inappropriateness
  - stability/lability
  - range, i.e. superficial/deep/blunted/theatrical.
- Comment on whether observed mood fits in with neurovegetative features.

Thoughts

- Speed
- Form (i.e. normal, circumstantial, tangential, loosening of association, incoherence, paralogical thinking, vagueness, neologisms – these are terms used to describe the organization of the person's thoughts.
- Content may be normal or delusional. Between these two extremes there may be magical thinking, overvalued ideas, or idiosyncratic ideas. These features will often be picked up during the course of the interview and confirmed in the MSE.

Table 9.2 continued

Perceptual disturbances
May be observed objectively during the clinical interview, or elicited in history: hallucinations, illusions (perceptual distortion of an existing stimulus). Perceptual disturbances may occur in any sensory modality.

Insight
May be full or partial or non-existent

Note: The patient's mental status is being assessed *throughout* the interview.

PART III
Management of specific mental health issues and disorders

10 Suicide and attempted suicide

'Suicide' and 'attempted suicide' should be viewed as two separate behaviours, each with its own causes and outcome, which overlap to a certain degree.

Suicide is defined as a wilful, self-inflicted, life-threatening act, which has resulted in death. *Attempted suicide* is a non-fatal act in which an individual causes self-injury by whatever means.

Nurses will face one of two situations, namely:
- patients who have suicidal ideas as part of the presentation (suicidal preoccupation may be elicited in the history, evaluation, systematic enquiry, or mental state examination and should always be enquired into); and
- patients who have survived a suicide attempt and need to be evaluated for the risk of potential suicide.

Patients need to be assessed for potential suicide. The nurse can use the Di Vasto ('SAD CHILDREN') Scale (1979), or any other similar tool that uses an acronym for easy recall and reference.

Evaluating the risk of suicide

'SAD CHILDREN': a suicide potential assessment scale

Nurses can use the 'SAD CHILDREN' acronym in many situations. For example, they can assess whether a patient is at risk for suicide and can plan interventions. None of the items below should be seen in isolation; instead, they should be seen contextually.

Table 10.1 Suicide potential assessment scale

S   Support system

Is there a support system for the patient? An absence of support for the patient increases the risk. Others also sometimes rely on the patient for support.

A   Alcohol

Does the patient use alcohol? Alcohol acts as a depressant. Many suicide attempts are made when patients are intoxicated.

Assault

Has the patient been raped, battered by a spouse, sexually abused, or experienced social upheavals such as moving, or a job change?

D   Depression

Is the patient in the early recovery stages of depression? This increases the risk of another suicide attempt as energy and drive begin to return to the patient.

Delusion

Does the patient suffer from paranoid delusions?

C   Communication

Has the patient communicated suicidal intentions, either directly or indirectly? Patients who communicate their intention to commit suicide give the nurse an opportunity to explore. Nurses should also be alert to indirect communication of intent, for example: 'I won't see you again.'

Changes in behaviour

Has there been a change in the patient's behaviour, such as writing a will, giving away prized possessions, cancelling social arrangements, or taking out extra insurance policies?

Table 10.1 continued

H Hostility
Does the patient express strong anger towards others that may result in a suicide attempt as a means of punishment?

History
Is there a history of previous suicide attempts? The more often the patient has attempted suicide, the greater the chances of eventual success. What methods have been used before? Patients with a history of high-lethal methods or patients who have changed the method from a low-lethal to a high-lethal method are at greater risk than those with a history of low-lethal methods. Family attempts at suicide are a risk factor. Have there been recurrent suicides or suicide attempts in the family?

Hallucinations
Does the patient hear command hallucinations, i.e. voices ordering the patient to commit suicide?

I Impulsiveness
Is the patient impulsive? The personality and coping skills of the patient during a crisis are significant since the impulsive person is a high suicide risk.

Illness
Does the patient have a chronic illness such as terminal cancer or has the patient recently been diagnosed with HIV, for example?

L Lethality
Has the patient chosen a high-lethal method to commit suicide? Is the patient aware of the lethality of the plan? Does the patient want to be rescued? Men tend to use more lethal methods such as hanging, shooting, or jumping, than women. The nurse should assess the client's awareness of the lethality of the plan to commit suicide and his desire to be rescued.

D Demography
Certain demographic factors increase the risk. Is the patient:
- living alone?
- recently divorced?
- in difficulty with a relationship?

Table 10.1 continued

- unemployed?
- in financial difficulty?
- in trouble with the police?
- female (suicide is attempted more often but is usually low-lethal)?

R	**Reaction of the evaluator**
	What is your reaction? The evaluator's subjective view may vary from anger to indifference or irritation. This is more common when patients have Axis II traits or an Axis II diagnosis. They can be antisocial, borderline cases, or histrionic. This subjective feeling by the evaluator could indicate that the patient is using the suicide threat to manipulate, which thus lessens the risk of suicide. Feeling empathy and a strong desire to care could indicate a higher risk of suicide.

E	**Events leading to the suicide attempt**
	Has the patient experienced significant lifestyle changes such as the loss or threatened loss of a significant other, examination failure, loss of a body part, or loss of a job or accommodation? The greater the loss, the greater the potential for suicide.

N	**No hope**
	Do you feel no hope? In extreme situations both nurse and patient may experience hopelessness.

Nurses should be doubly alert when patients who have verbalized suicidal intent suddenly 'cheer up' or say that they are no longer suicidal (even where external circumstances and factors could account for the change). These patients may well have resolved to act on the suicidal idea. Note that the presence of any of the psychiatric disorders listed in Table 10.2 markedly increase risk.

Admission to hospital is indicated for treatment of the underlying condition. Improvement in depressive symptoms may be associated with a paradoxical increased risk of suicide.

Table 10.2 Psychiatric disorders that carry an increased risk of suicide

---

- Major depression (including psychotic depression)
- Bipolar mood disorder (either manic or depressed)
- Schizophrenia
- Panic disorder
- Antisocial personality disorder: increased risk of suicide
- Borderline personality disorder: increased risk of suicide and attempted suicide
- Substance abuse (alcohol/cannabis/mandrax/cocaine/benzodiazepines)

Never rely on a patient's word that he or she will not commit suicide.

Psychiatric disorders

There are a number of psychiatric disorders associated with suicide. Some are more common at different ages and this should be taken into account when evaluating the patient.

Young adults (15 to 25)

There are various risk factors that may feature in this age group.

Drug and alcohol abuse

Any of the street drugs may cause depression, including cannabis (dagga), mandrax, and cocaine.

Personality disorder

There is an increased risk of suicide and attempted suicide in males with antisocial personality disorder. Females with borderline personality disorder are at risk for attempted suicide.

Relationship difficulties

Young adults who have relationship difficulties with either parents or loved ones are at risk.

Bipolar mood disorder

Both the manic and depressed forms of this disorder are associated with a higher suicide risk. A family history of suicide may indicate the presence of bipolar mood disorder.

Schizophrenia

The onset of this disorder is in late adolescence and early adulthood and suicide is common in the early stages of the disease, especially among young men (up to 10 per cent of schizophrenics kill themselves).

The middle-aged and elderly

The incidence of psychiatric disorder increases with increasing age. The following disorders are common.

Alcohol abuse

Alcohol abuse increases the risk of suicide among patients in this age group.

Bipolar mood disorder

Bipolar mood disorder in the middle-aged and elderly increases the risk of suicide.

Major depression

There is a high risk for suicide among patients who suffer from major depression.

Chronic illness or pain

Illness that carries a social stigma, for example HIV, could precipitate suicide. Chronic pain should be treated aggressively by referring the patient to a physician or pain clinic.

Nursing interventions

After a suicide attempt always try to assess whether the patient is still in severe stress. If so, there is a risk of a repeat attempt.

Table 10.3 Risk factors for suicide

- Elderly male
- Psychiatric disorder
- Chronic illness (HIV/AIDS, especially young people; and cancer, diabetes, etc. especially older people)
- Relationship difficulties (parent/child relationship problems, especially young people, and divorce/death of a spouse, especially older people)
- Chronic pain
- Previous suicide attempt
- Choice of lethal method
- Hopelessness

Intervene immediately by following these guidelines:

- Don't minimize the attempt or its significance. Be honest with the patient. Discuss the situation. When you make a referral, explain the value of long-term treatment.
- Help relieve the patient's stress. For example, if the patient is in a semi-private room, be sure the roommate is compatible. Allow the patient to smoke, if desired. If the patient enjoys TV or the radio, make sure these are available.
- Don't do anything that the patient might interpret as punishment. Make sure any physical restraints are for the patient's protection and not just for your convenience.
- Help the patient set goals to relieve the unbearable stress that precipitated the suicide attempt. But be careful. Don't solve problems for the patient.
- Help re-build self-respect. If the condition permits, encourage the patient to participate in his or her care.
- Maintain good nutrition. If the patient won't eat three well-balanced meals a day, provide nutritious snacks instead. The patient may eat more if finger foods, such as sandwiches, chicken, and fruit are provided.
- Don't make careless remarks, especially around a semi-comatose patient. The patient, other nurses, or the family may overhear them, causing unnecessary embarrassment.
- Don't leave your patient alone. Never let the patient leave your floor without an attendant. Encourage family

members to keep the patient company. Many hospitals hire people especially to stay with suicidal patients.
- Protect the patient. Remove any potentially lethal articles from the room. Watch what visitors bring.
- Try to treat your patient as you would any other. If you pity suicidal patients, they may resent it. If you're too accommodating, patients may feel they don't deserve the attention. If you're insecure or defensive with them, they probably won't trust your judgement.

Dealing with the family

Family members and friends may respond to a loved one's suicide attempt in the following ways:
- They may try to forget the attempt.
- They usually avoid discussing the attempt because they don't know what to say.
- The attempt may have scared, embarrassed, or puzzled them.
- They may feel guilty because they failed to detect their loved one's crisis.
- When they do discuss the attempt, they do so awkwardly, which only compounds the patient's stress.

The nurse should:
- teach the family about the patient's condition;
- make sure the family understands that release from the hospital does not mean that the problems are over; and
- make sure that the patient has support; patients need someone they trust, as well as someone who accepts and cares for them. Without this support, there is still a suicide risk.

Dealing with your feelings

Nurses should not allow their own attitudes towards suicide to intrude on the quality of care:

- Nurses who see suicide as a character weakness may be impatient with, and perhaps show disdain for, the patient. They may also focus on physical problems and ignore emotional ones. They should avoid both reactions and try to be as understanding as possible.
- Nurses who view suicide as an emotional illness may try to resolve the patient's distress themselves. Instead they should direct patients to professional help.

Medical treatment

The following basic principles apply when treating suicidal individuals:

- Admit patients who are at high risk for suicide.
- Treat the underlying psychiatric disorder.
- Address the psychosocial problems.
- Treat all medical problems.
- Give electroconvulsive therapy to suicidal patients with severe depression or psychotic depression as it acts more quickly than antidepressants.
- Admit borderline personality disorder patients who are in crisis and become suicidal, but only for a short period (one to three days) to get over the crisis. Discharge them as soon as possible. Borderline patients who remain in hospital for long periods tend to become dependent on psychiatric facilities.
- Patients who are suicidal as a result of severe psychosocial stressors such as divorce or financial difficulty, may benefit from short-term admission and sedation followed by brief supportive psychotherapy aimed at helping them come to terms with the problem. It is helpful to identify practical solutions (for example seeing the bank manager or seeking alternative employment) and support systems such as family, friends, and a minister of religion.
- Short-term sedation may be used in extremely suicidal individuals for a day or two to see them over a crisis situation:
  - clothiapine (Etomine) 40–80 mg (intramuscularly or orally) eight-hourly as required, either in combination

with diazepam 5 mg orally daily as required or oxazepam 10mg orally three times a day or lorazepam orally 2–4 mg two to three times a day. (The aim is to keep the patient lightly sedated.)

- Drugs that have been found to exacerbate suicidal thoughts are: Noradrenergic re-uptake inhibitors, especially maprotiline; and benzodiazepines, especially alprazolam (Xanor).
- Drugs that have been found to either reduce or have a neutral effect on suicidal thoughts are:
  - Serotonin re-uptake inhibitors, namely fluoxetine (Prozac), paroxetine (Aropax), citalopram (Cipramil), and clomipramine (Anafranil).
  - flupenthixol depot (Fluanxol) 20 mg administered intramuscularly once a month may also be useful, particularly with personality disorders.

Crisis intervention

If a patient is described as being in crisis it means that he or she is facing a problem that cannot easily be resolved with coping mechanisms that have worked previously. Hospitalization, planned surgery, loss of health or limbs, pressure of work, loss of employment, rape, or threatened loss of life are all examples of events that could precipitate a crisis situation. Crisis intervention implies providing the immediate aid that the patient requires to regain equilibrium.

- The *short-term* goal is the psychological resolution of the individual's immediate crisis and restoration to at least the previous level of functioning, or to an even better level than before the crisis.
- The *long-term* goal is personality growth.

A crisis must be handled within twenty-four hours. A trained nurse can do this. Effective crisis management will prevent the development of psychopathology in the patient and the need for psychiatric treatment later on.

11 Crisis and victims of violence

The steps of crisis management

Step 1: Establish a trust relationship

During this phase nurses should present themselves to their patients as being able to offer help. Closeness plays an important role. It provides security for the patient and shows that the nurse really cares. Instil hope in patients so that they believe that they can come out of the situation successfully.

The nurse must show genuine interest in, and respect for, the patient. The nurse should demonstrate an attitude of warmth, empathy, and acceptance, so that the patient feels totally at ease.

Step 2: Assessment

Identify the precipitating event. Was it an accident, rape, the diagnosis of an incurable disease, infidelity in marriage, dismissal from work, or the sudden death of a loved one or family member? Establish to what extent the crisis interferes with the patient's daily activities. For example, is there an insurance policy available in the event of the death of a breadwinner? Is there money available for rent, petrol, or food? Is someone available to take care of the daily chores?

Evaluate the person's support structures, such as family, friends, church, pastor, or doctor, and assess how rapidly they could be mobilized. Identify what influence the event has had on the patient. Even in this early stage of evaluation you should carefully consider ways of developing the patient's coping mechanisms. It is important to determine whether the patient takes any drugs or other substances. Assess for suicidal risk!

Step 3: Planning

After a thorough evaluation of all aspects, the nurse and the patient should look at alternative solutions and evaluate them. Remember that in the process of a crisis the nurse often needs to take a more direct approach, as the patient is in a state of disequilibrium.

The following aspects should be attended to:

- How long has the patient been in crisis?
- How much has the crisis already influenced his or her daily functioning, lifestyle, or routine?
- What sources of aid are available to the patient?
- What problem-solving mechanisms does the patient usually employ?
- Has he or she already tried them? Did this help?
- What else is available?

Step 4: Intervention

This phase consists of a specific, structured, mutually agreed-upon intervention to mobilize the patient's support systems and other aid. For example, the patient could consult with family members, the doctor, or a pastor to shed more light on the problem. Interventions could be implemented to change the patient's perceptions and reactions as a result of his or her experience and belief system. For example, a patient's mother could perhaps be asked to look after the children in the afternoons.

The patient must be guided toward an intellectual understanding of the crisis. Patients often fail to see any connection between the events in their lives and the pain that they are experiencing at present. In counselling the patient, focus on the errors of thought that a patient makes with regard to his or her experience of the crisis. Nurses should make patients aware of the fact that their emotional reaction to the crisis is excessive and inappropriate and that they should develop alternative thought patterns to counter similar crises.

These alternative thought patterns give the patient a new perception of stress and increase self-knowledge, while also offering useful coping mechanisms and an opportunity for personality growth.

Step 5: Follow-up

Follow-up with the patient after the initial crisis management is an integral part of the treatment. In this way the nurse can determine whether the patient has worked through the crisis successfully. If not, the person will react in the same way in similar crises and personality growth will not take place.

Victims of violence/trauma

Trauma refers to situations in which a person is rendered powerless and great danger is involved. Trauma in this sense refers to events involving death or injury or the possibility of death and injury. These events must be unusual and out of the ordinary, not events that are part of the normal course of life. Trauma encompasses events of such intensity or magnitude of horror that they would overwhelm anybody's usual ability to cope.

The rape survivor

Caring for a rape survivor immediately after the event won't be easy, no matter how well you are prepared. But do your best. She'll need your understanding to relieve her profound distress and possibly prevent crisis.

As you begin your assessment, be careful of what you say and do. Don't intensify a crisis in your patient. Try to appear calm but not indifferent. Let the patient know that you share her horror of what's happened and that you won't brush it off as 'just another emergency'.

Encourage the patient to talk about it. But be prepared to listen, no matter how difficult that may be. Take what she says seriously, even if her story has inconsistencies. A rape survivor may be so disorientated that her first account of the assault doesn't make sense.

Don't criticize her – or let anyone else criticize her – for the way she acts and talks. The shock of rape may cause her to behave strangely. At various times during the initial assessment and the doctor's examination, you can expect some or all of these shock-related signs:

- inconsistencies in her story;
- incoherent speech;
- confusion about numbers;
- inability to determine time intervals;
- crying, with periods of uncontrollable sobbing;
- restlessness or tenseness;
- inappropriate smiling or laughing; and
- extreme anger, accompanied by wishes of revenge.

Occasionally, patients may hide their extreme stress under an unusually calm, composed exterior. When this happens, watch closely. No matter how calmly the patient relates the details of her assault, never let anyone refuse to take her seriously. Instead, try to estimate her internal stress level; it may be greater than that of the patient who shows her distress.

Encourage trust

Do your best to establish a trusting relationship. Tell the patient your name, if you haven't done so already, and reassure her that you'll stay with her during the examination. Try to assess her level of understanding, then use words and terms she knows. If you find this difficult, ask yourself whether you're hiding behind professional jargon and technical terms to cope with your own feelings. Try to find another way to cope. Remember, you add to the patient's distress by making her feel ignorant.

Does your patient seem uncooperative or hostile? Try to be understanding. Consider what may be causing these reactions.

For example, ask yourself:
- What exactly happened during the assault?
- How does this patient perceive the rape?
- How is she coping with it? Does she think she's to blame for the attack?
- Are her usual support systems available to her? If not, are they unavailable because of her specific reactions or attitudes toward rape?
- Has the patient received adequate emotional support from you and other health care professionals?
- Have you and others tried to preserve the patient's dignity and prevent further humiliation?

Supply needs

Take her to a private area. Try to find out what your patient really wants. Expectations may vary depending on her perception of the rape. For example, does she primarily seek physical care, police intervention, or emotional support? She may want all three, but one will take top priority.

To determine this, listen carefully and show your concern. Ask: 'How can I help you most?' If she feels threatened by others in the emergency department, try to find some privacy. Then encourage her to talk, so you can accurately assess her balancing factors (i.e. her usual coping mechanisms and the strengths that may help her through difficult situations).

The physical examination

When you've completed your initial assessment, prepare the patient for the physical examination. Before you do, assess her psychological ability to tolerate a pelvic examination at this time. *The additional stress may trigger repeat flashes of the rape and precipitate a crisis.*

To prepare the patient for the physical examination, you should do the following:
- Find out first whether she's ever had such an examination. Remember, she may not have, particularly if she's under the age of twenty.
- Explain exactly what it involves, why it must be performed, and what is expected of her.

- Go over each step carefully, repeating your explanation if necessary.
- Encourage her to ask all the questions she wants answered before proceeding further. Answer honestly and reassuringly.
- Urge her to relax, if she can, to make the examination easier.

12 Mentally-challenged individuals and mental illness

There is a substantial overlap between the treatment of mental illness and the treatment of mentally-challenged individuals because psychiatric disorders are more prevalent in the mentally challenged than in the general population. The reasons for this may be organic, social, or a combination of both. Consequently, those working in the field of mental illness need to be thoroughly familiar with treating mentally-challenged individuals.

Terminology

Different countries use different terms. Currently 'mentally challenged' is the term preferred in South Africa, while 'mental retardation' is the generally accepted term in the USA. In the UK, the term 'learning disability' has replaced mental handicap, but this may cause confusion when mentally-challenged children need to be distinguished from those with reading or writing difficulties.

Definition and diagnosis

An individual is diagnosed as mentally-challenged when all three of the following conditions, which are based on the definition of the American Association of Mental Retardation (1992), are present:

- significantly sub-average intellectual functioning (an IQ < 70);
- related limitations in two or more of the following applicable adaptive skill areas:
  - communication;
  - self-care;
  - home-living;
  - social skills;
  - community use;
  - self-direction;
  - health and safety;
  - functional academics;
  - leisure;
  - work; and
- onset before age eighteen.

Classification

The classification of intellectual impairment is set out in Table 12.1. A second classification is used in an educational context (Table 12.2).

Table 12.1 Classification of intellectual impairment according to severity

DSM-IV code	Range of IQ Score	Developmental characteristics
317 Mild	50–55 to 70	Socially competent; may need guidance and assistance during period of stress.
318.0 Moderate	35–40 to 50–55	Basic self-care skills; need some supervision and guidance.

Table 12.1 continued

318.1 Severe	20–25 to 35–40	Some self-care skills; need full supervision.
318.2 Profound	Below 20–25	Minimal self-care skills; need constant nursing care.

Source: Adapted from American Psychiatric Association, 1994. *Diagnostic and statistical manual of mental disorders.* 4th edn. Washington D.C: The American Psychiatric Association.

Table 12.2 Education classification

Classification	Range of IQ score	School of placement
Educable	50 to 70	Special class in a regular school
Trainable	25 to 60	Special school
Special care	Below 30	Special care centre

Note: There is a move towards progressive mainstreaming of mentally challenged children in South Africa.

Source: Adapted from American Psychiatric Association, 1994. *Diagnostic and statistical manual of mental disorders.* 4th edn. Washington, DC: The American Psychiatric Association.

Prevalence

Approximately 80 per cent of mentally-challenged individuals fall within the mild (IQ 50 to 70) range. Prevalence rates are as follows:
- 3 per cent of population – IQ < 70
- 4 per 1 000 – IQ < 50
- 1 per 1 000 – IQ < 30

Aetiology

Determining the causes of intellectual impairment depends on the medical history, including the family history, a physical examination, and where indicated, special investigations. Causes are usually classified according to the timing of their onset.

- *Prenatal* causes occur from the time of conception to the onset of labour.
- *Perinatal* causes occur during labour and delivery of the infant.
- *Postnatal* causes occur after the first week of life.
- *Idiopathic* cases are those in which no plausible cause can be identified. (When an adequate history, examination, or special investigations are not available, the cause is considered to be unknown.)

Most mildly mentally-challenged individuals are idiopathic cases. In some instances familial (polygenic) or environmental factors are implicated. In moderate, severe, and profound cases (IQ < 50) the causes are more often due to organic brain damage (Table 12.3).

Table 12.3 Aetiology of mental challenges

Prenatal 45%
Chromosomal abnormalities:
- Down's syndrome
- Other

Inherited metabolic disorders
Dysmorphic syndromes
Congenital abnormalities of the brain
Other familial disorders
Acquired diseases during pregnancy

Perinatal 15%
Prematurity and its complications
Full-term asphyxia

Table 12.3 continued

Postnatal 15%
Infections, e.g. meningitis, encephalitis.
Trauma:
- Accidental
- Non-accidental

Other illnesses during childhood

Idiopathic (unknown) 25%

Source: Adapted from American Psychiatric Association. 1994.
Diagnostic and statistical manual of mental disorders. 4th edn.
Washington, DC: The American Psychiatric Association.

Management

Management of children and adults will be dealt with separately.

Children

Principles
- The aim is to achieve the full developmental potential and maximum social integration for each child.
- Development consists of progressive, coherent changes in skills and abilities. Each phase is important and intervention can never start too early.
- Children develop best in a family setting.

Practice
The following practical guidelines need to be applied:
- The parents must be approached sensitively when they are told about their child's condition.
- The parents need support, either by a professional or in lay groups.

- Parents should be given genetic counselling where indicated.
- There should be a screening programme in community health clinics so that children suspected of being mentally-challenged can be referred to a developmental clinic for assessment and management.
- Developmental intervention must be introduced to ensure optimal development and preparation for school.
- Appropriate school placement in:
  - a special class if the child is mildly mentally-challenged;
  - a special school if the child is moderately mentally-challenged; and
  - a special care centre if the child is severely or profoundly mentally-challenged.

Most children will live at home. Admission to a residential facility or hospital is indicated only when:
- a court finds that a child is in need of care;
- the home is either unsafe or unsatisfactory; and/or
- the child requires treatment because of medical or behavioural complications.

Adults

Principles

The principles applied here are as follows:
- The aim is to achieve maximal personal growth, social integration, and autonomy.
- Where possible, mentally-challenged individuals should live in the community. This concept is not limited to physical presence in the community, but also implies social relationships and valued community participation.
- Each individual has a right to economic security and a decent standard of living. This includes the opportunity to work or engage in other meaningful occupations.
- Although community care is the ideal, there are individuals who will have to be hospitalized in the long term owing to the nature or extent of the mental challenges, their behavioural characteristics, or lack of suitable family with whom they can be placed.

Residential options include:
- care in the home if the family can cope;
- a group home in the community with suitable supervision; or
- care in hospital if the person has medical or nursing needs.

Occupational options are:
- open labour for some mildly mentally-challenged people;
- sheltered employment for those able to maintain at least 50 per cent productivity;
- a protective workshop for those who are less than 50 per cent productive; or
- an activity for the severely and profoundly mentally-challenged.

Most adults living in the community will have their medical needs met in the primary health setting. The support and attention of the multidisciplinary team may be required for the management of psychiatric complications.

13 Mood disorders

Major depressive disorder is one of the most common psychiatric disturbances in adulthood. The prevalence of this disorder is 15 per cent, and that of bipolar disorder 1 per cent. Only 50 per cent of people suffering from depression receive treatment for it. In 50 per cent of these cases, the treatment is inadequate because of insufficient dosage of antidepressant, or low compliance.

There are many misconceptions regarding depression. One of the myths about depression is that depression and sadness are the same thing. The fact is that we all feel sad or unhappy from time to time, but often we know the cause, and our reaction is understandable. This sadness usually disappears once the cause of the emotion has been removed – unlike the persistent sadness associated with depression.

Depression can sometimes also present as body pains. Patients may complain of body pains and not of feelings of sadness. Clinicians should be alert to this possibility and exclude physical causes before diagnosing depression.

Causes of depression

Depression is a complex illness. It is not caused by any single factor, but can be triggered by several chemically-related, psychological, or physical factors. It would seem that depressive episodes occur because of changes (in neurons and neurotransmitters) in the brain.

Other causes of depression include:

- side-effects of prescribed drugs such as tranquillizers, sleeping pills, appetite suppressants, stimulants, and antihypertensives; and
- certain medical conditions such as anaemia, an underactive thyroid gland, and viral infections.

Age of onset, natural history treated and untreated

Depressive disorder

Of note in this disorder is that:

- 50 per cent of patients experience the first episode before the age of forty;
- untreated, the duration of a depressive episode is between six and twelve months;
- with treatment, the duration is three months;
- with increase in age, episodes are more frequent and of longer duration; and
- 5 to 10 per cent of patients with major depression may have a manic episode at some later stage.

Bipolar disorder (see p. 150)

In this disorder:

- patients usually experience depressive and manic episodes;
- 10 to 20 per cent have only manic episodes;
- onset usually coincides with a depressive episode (in 75 per cent of female patients and 67 per cent of male patients);
- mania develops rapidly (within hours or days);
- untreated mania will last for approximately three months; and
- some patients have 'rapid cycling' (short, repetitive episodes) – this pattern is more common in females.

The case study below highlights the symptoms of depression as a nurse would be likely to encounter them in the field.

Mrs. X is a forty-year-old woman who is employed as a secretary at a primary school. She visited her family doctor complaining of sleeplessness, poor appetite, and weight loss. Her symptoms had begun two months earlier when she was admitted to hospital for a previous neck injury. The injury was not serious but she was experiencing neck pain and was unable to work for several weeks. She found this distressing, since she had been working at this school for fifteen years and was convinced that her employer would replace her. She was unable to occupy herself at home.

Shortly after her admission to hospital, she began to have difficulty in sleeping. She would awaken at 4 am and be awake for the next two hours thinking about things she had done wrong in the past. She became particularly preoccupied with the fact that she had had a premarital sexual relationship with a school friend. Although she had already discussed this matter with her husband, she felt she should confess it to her minister. Her husband tried to reassure her and said that he had no concern about what had happened, but she could not be persuaded. Her appetite diminished and she lost approximately 4 kg over a period of two months. Finally, she sought out her minister and, with great anxiety, explained her concern about the premarital sexual relationship. Despite his comforting and understanding response, she continued to worry about her 'sin'. She began telling her husband and children that she was a worthless and evil person and that they would be much better off without her.

She steadily lost interest in all her favourite recreational activities, which had included tennis and reading.

During the week before she went to see her family doctor, she became increasingly anxious and restless, paced around, and felt unable to sit still. Her feelings of guilt increased. When her family asked her what she had done that was so terribly wrong, she replied vaguely that it was too terrible to discuss with 'decent people'. She also made more references to the fact that 'everyone would be better off without her'.

On evaluation, the family doctor observed a plump, un-kempt woman with an expression of anguish and misery on her face. She described herself as feeling extremely sad, anxious, and pessimistic. She burst into tears several times as she described her 'sin' of the premarital sexual relation-ship. She described herself as being overwhelmed with feel-ings of guilt, worthlessness, and hopelessness. She twisted her hands almost continuously and nervously played with her hair. She stated that her family would be better off without her and that she had been considering taking her life by shooting herself. She felt that after death she would go to hell, where she would experience eternal torment, but that this would be a just punishment for her 'sin'.

Five years prior to this illness, the patient had had a similar episode, which her family described as 'virtually identical'. She was hospitalized at that time, treated with antidepressant medication (amitriptyline), and responded well. She had recovered fully and become her usual self, with no signs of mental illness during the intervening years. The family described her two episodes of depression as some-thing 'quite different' from her usual self.

This patient was treated with tricyclic antidepressant medication. She improved markedly within three weeks and returned home to resume her usual routine.

There are two basic symptoms in mood disorders, one for depression and one for mania (see p. 150). Depressive episodes can occur in both major depressive disorders and bipolar disorder.

Some patients with bipolar disorder have mixed states with both manic and depressive features, or seem to experience brief episodes of depression during manic episodes. These episodes can last for anything between a few minutes and a few hours.

Depressive episode

The key symptoms are:
• depressed mood most of the day and nearly every day;

- subjective rapport or observation; and
- loss of interest or pleasure in all or most activities.

The other symptoms of which not all need to be present during the same two-week period are:
- Neurovegetative signs including:
  - weight loss or gain;
  - appetite increase or decrease;
  - insomnia or hypersomnia;
  - abnormal menstrual cycle;
  - diminished concentration, memory problems, or indecisiveness; and
  - sexual dysfunction.
- General signs including:
  - fatigue or loss of energy;
  - recurrent thoughts about death and suicidal thoughts;
  - feelings of worthlessness or excessive guilt, which may be inappropriate and excessive (delusional);
  - headaches and general body pains; and
  - psychomotor agitation or retardation.

Patients often have the following complaints that should lead the clinician to consider depression:
- general body pains;
- the whole body being 'sore' or 'weak';
- pains starting at the patient's feet and extending to the top of the head;
- scratching inside the top of the head;
- bewitchments and fear of death;
- hearing voices calling or speaking and 'thwasa'; and
- snakes in the patient's stomach.

In depression, the physical examination and basic medical screening tests will usually be normal despite these complaints.

Depression causes clinically significant distress or impairment in social, occupational, or other important areas of functioning. Possible physiological effects of a substance or effects of a general medical condition must be excluded. The symptoms are not better accounted for by bereavement.

Patients presenting with major depression should also be asked about episodes of mania or cyclothymia in themselves or in blood relations.

Manic episodes

See p. 150 for manic disorders.

Dysthymic and cyclothymic episodes

These episodes are characterized by the presence of mood symptoms that are less severe than the symptoms of major depressive disorder and of mania in bipolar disorder.

Complicated depression

Depression may occur with psychotic features that are usually congruent with the mood. These include:
- thought disorder;
- delusions;
- hallucinations; and
- loss of insight.

Complicated depression is a severe disease and the prognosis is poor. The condition is treated with antipsychotic drugs in addition to antidepressants and may require electroconvulsive therapy (ECT).

Coexisting disorders with mood disorders

Mood disorders may be accompanied by:
- anxiety;
- alcohol dependence;

- other substance-related disorders; and
- medical conditions.

Complications

The most serious complication is the possibility of suicide. On the social and personal level the complications are:
- poor performance at school and at work;
- marital discord (decreased sexual interest); and
- drug and alcohol abuse.

Remember to use the 'SAD CHILDREN' acronym to assess suicidal risk (see Chapter 10).

Treatment of depression

Antidepressant medication is probably the most important advancement in treating depression. Most people suffering from depression find the combination of psychotherapy and antidepressants practical and highly effective. (If there is a history of mania or a family history of bipolar disorder, great caution must be exercised in prescribing antidepressants: start low, go slow, watch carefully for mania, and possibly prescribe lithium in conjunction with the antidepressant). For a treatment outline see Figure 13.1

Nursing management of depression

When to refer or hospitalize
Hospitalization or referral should be considered in cases where:
- there is a suicide or homicide risk;
- treatment has failed;
- there is a need for diagnostic procedures;
- there are rapidly progressing symptoms and failure of the patient's usual support system; and

- a patient's ability to care for himself or herself is grossly reduced.

Notes

- Specific serotonin re-uptake inhibitors (SSRIs) such as fluoxetine, paroxetine, and citalopram have fewer side-effects, are effective and non-toxic, and some generics may be available, but may be more expensive than generic TCAs.
- Tricyclic antidepressants (TCAs) are contra-indicated in heart disease and are toxic in overdose (amitriptyline, imipramine).
- Before changing medication establish whether:
  - there has been sufficient patient compliance;
  - dosage has been adequate; and
  - treatment has been of adequate duration.
- If the patient has been taking a TCA, change to an SSRI. If the patient has already been using an SSRI, try a different SSRI before changing to a TCA.

Counselling of patient and family

Listen, using effective and therapeutic communication. Once you have identified clear signs of depression, discuss referral to a psychologist or psychiatrist with the patient and then refer him or her. However, if there is a serious risk that the person may commit suicide (e.g. the person seems to have planned or thought of ways to commit suicide) they should be sent straight to the hospital casualty. Make sure they are accompanied by a responsible person.

- Ask about risk of suicide. Has the patient often thought of death or dying? Does the patient have a specific suicide plan? Has he or she made serious suicide attempts in the past? Can the patient be sure not to act on suicidal ideas? Close supervision by family or friends, or hospitalization may be needed. Ask about risk of harm to others.
- Plan short-term activities, which give the patient enjoyment or build confidence.
- Encourage the patient to resist pessimism and self-criticism, not to act on pessimistic ideas (e.g. ending

Figure 13.1 Treatment outline for depression

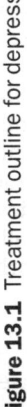

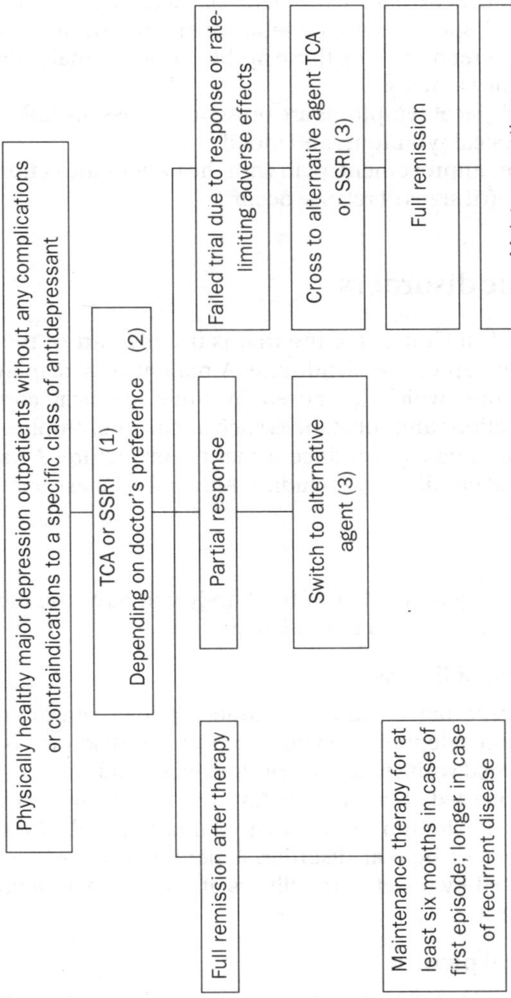

Physically healthy major depression outpatients without any complications or contraindications to a specific class of antidepressant

TCA or SSRI (1)
Depending on doctor's preference (2)

Full remission after therapy

Partial response

Failed trial due to response or rate-limiting adverse effects

Switch to alternative agent (3)

Cross to alternative agent TCA or SSRI (3)

Maintenance therapy for at least six months in case of first episode; longer in case of recurrent disease

Full remission

Maintenance therapy

marriage, leaving job), and not to concentrate on negative or guilty thoughts.
- Identify current life problems or social stresses. Focus on small, specific steps patients might take towards reducing or better managing these problems. Avoid major decisions or life changes.
- If physical symptoms are present, discuss the link between physical symptoms and mood.
- After improvement, plan with the patient the action to be taken if signs of relapse occur.

Manic disorders

Mania is a clinical picture that is usually part of the bipolar (manic depressive) syndrome. A patient may display manic behaviour, which is caused by other medical conditions. Medications and substances such as cocaine, amphetamines, and steroids can produce a maniform picture. A variety of medical conditions, including Aids, may be associated with mania.

History

Commonly a member of the family will have the condition, (especially a first-degree relative).

Pattern of illness

The onset may occur at any time in adolescent or adult life. The manic depressive syndrome (bipolar disorder) is usually associated with somewhat prolonged periods of being manic or depressed. Mania may last for weeks or months and depression for months or years. Mania can be the first clinical evidence of bipolar disorder. A poorer prognosis is usually indicated by onset of the illness at an early age (teens, early twenties).

Clinical picture

The onset usually occurs over some weeks. A very acute onset within hours or a day or so, raises the suspicion of other causes, especially drugs. A medical cause should be suspected in a patient over the age of forty, particularly if the onset is either sudden, or a first manic episode.

The following may be evident:

- *Mood* becomes elated and/or irritable and there may be associated aggression.
- *Motor behaviour* is increased, and the person is very active and tends to talk incessantly.
- *Judgement* is usually impaired and the individual becomes involved in situations that could have serious adverse consequences. Unfavourable business deals, spending sprees, gambling, and drinking are examples.
- *Thinking* is rapid. The patient is easily distracted and may move from one topic to another, often making clang (rhyming) associations and puns.
- *Inhibition* decreases and there is an inability to assess social occasions appropriately.
- *Social intrusiveness* in these individuals generally becomes a problem.
- *Interpersonal relationships* become strained and insight is impaired.
- *Sleep* is disturbed and may be absent in serious manic states.
- *Sexual activity* is usually increased.
- *Eating* becomes erratic and there is a trend towards weight loss; the total intake of food and drink usually decreases.
- *Sensory awareness* may be heightened.
- *Insight* is totally lost as mania becomes worse, and there may be grandiose delusions and hallucinations. Paranoid delusions may occur at this stage, but are short-lived, as are the hallucinations.
- *Conversations* become difficult or impossible and such a patient may be difficult to interrupt.

Hospitalization may be difficult as they 'have never felt better'. Usually, the family has never felt worse and they are often exhausted and 'battered' by the patient. It is extremely important to contact a family member or informant if mania is suspected!

Management

As patients generally have impaired insight and usually have a feeling of well-being it may be very difficult to persuade them to be hospitalized. *There should be very sound reasons for not hospitalizing a manic patient.* The serious damage that a manic patient may cause to him or herself or to family must be an overriding consideration. If a patient is not prepared to consent to voluntary admission, the *Mental Health Act* may be invoked in order to detain such an individual.

The cornerstone of treatment of mania is the use of antipsychotic medication (neuroleptics). Doses will usually have to be fairly high in a highly aroused, very overactive patient. Haloperidol in doses from 5 mg to 20 mg daily may be required to bring about rapid control of over-activity, agitation, and aggression. Haloperidol can be given intravenously, IMI, or orally in divided doses. Should the patient still be difficult, the addition of a benzodiazepine such as diazepam, can be considered. Intravenous administration of diazepam must be carefully managed as respiratory arrest can occur. Diazepam is extremely well absorbed by mouth and is very safe. Clonazepam may be useful to control some manic patients, but it is expensive. Lorazepam 2–4 mg orally or IV has proved effective in combination with haloperidol.

Even if the patient is to be transferred to a mental hospital, a neuroleptic will be required to facilitate the move. Electroconvulsive therapy may be used in difficult, unresponsive patients.

The long-term treatment for mania and also for bipolar disorder is lithium carbonate, for both its prophylactic and therapeutic effects. It is a useful medication in the prevention of illness in both mania and depression. Lithium should not be used in conjunction with *high* doses of neuroleptics (in excess of 40 mg of haloperidol per day). Lithium blood levels must be monitored and should run between 0.4 mmol/L and 1 mmol/L. Levels between 0.6 and 0.7 mmol/L are generally satisfactory. A number of anticonvulsants have been used instead of lithium, the best tested being sodium valproate. This should be used where lithium has failed, or where the patient has demonstrated intolerance of lithium, or there are other contraindications to its use. The unavailability of a blood-monitoring facility may limit the use of lithium. Lithium levels may rise dangerously if the patient becomes dehydrated or uses diuretics. Lithium can be thyrotoxic.

Management of the patient and family in general constitutes an important part of the approach. Remember that female bipolar patients have a very significant risk of having an attack during the puerperium. This has hazards for child and mother. Because of sexual arousal, the risk of pregnancy during a manic attack must be considered.

Prognosis

Bipolar disorder, especially with manic dominance, is a very serious illness. There is a risk of suicide and of early death due to other causes. The patient's capacity to work and relate to others may be significantly impaired.

The patient should be seen at least once by an expert who can advise on management, and thereafter expert advice should still be available. Genetic counselling must be considered. Poor compliance with treatment is not uncommon.

Nursing management

With manic patients, the nurse should be calm and relaxed, but firm, particularly when communicating limits.

Promote safety

- Provide a safe environment by reducing environmental stimuli. This can entail a quiet environment and a room where unnecessary items are removed.
- Ask the family to reduce the noise stimulation (low lighting can also help).

Monitor medication

Hyperactive and agitated behaviour responds to antipsychotics such as chlorpromazine and haloperidol. These medications are often used to help manage manic patients, who have started on lithium, as lithium takes one to two weeks to become effective.

Nursing interventions include monitoring patients for adverse side-effects of antipsychotic medications. See Chapter 25 for management of side-effects and a patient teaching plan for lithium (Table 25.4).

Promote reality based thinking

- Present reality by spending time with the patient.
- Do not appear to be in a hurry.
- Identify yourself, the time, the day, and other orienting information as needed.
- Behave consistently as this is reassuring to patients with altered thought processes.

Note: It is fruitless to argue, or try to reason with, delusional patients. This serves to harden the belief system and can impair development of trust. Remember to give positive reinforcement when patients focus on reality.

Set limits

Out of control, manipulative behaviour often requires limit setting. Patients should be managed in a firm and consistent manner, according to set limits. All staff members should agree on the limits.

Improve self-care

Personal hygiene and self-care is needed to ensure self-esteem and healthy social interactions. Hyperactive patients who are unwilling or unable to bathe, brush their teeth, shave, wash their hair, or change their clothes should be assisted by their family, or, if their self-care has deteriorated badly, admitted to hospital where they can be assisted by nurses.

Promote rest and sleep

Patients in the manic phase appear deceptively energetic when they may actually be nearing the point of exhaustion:

- Monitor them closely for signs of fatigue, and educate the family to make sure that the patient takes sufficient rest.

- Encourage and assist the patient to sleep more.
- Promote rest by decreasing light and noise, and by encouraging quiet activities.

14 Anxiety disorders

Anxiety is a normal response that may enhance performance. Anxiety *disorders*, however, are characterized by marked distress or by impairment in academic, occupational, or social functioning. The morbidity and mortality of anxiety disorders has been significantly underestimated in the past.

Anxiety disorders are typically under-diagnosed in primary care practice. Anxiety disorders should therefore be strongly considered in the differential diagnosis of a variety of physical and psychiatric symptoms. As anxiety disorders commonly lead to substance abuse and depression, underlying anxiety should be considered in all patients who abuse substances or manifest depression.

The most important step after having recognized the presence of pathological anxiety is to make a specific diagnosis, as there is a specific treatment for each anxiety disorder. The anxiety disorders include panic disorder, obsessive-compulsive disorder, social phobia, specific phobia, post-traumatic stress disorder, generalized anxiety disorder, and anxiety disorder due to a general medical condition.

Panic disorder

Panic disorder is characterized by panic attacks in the form of discrete periods of intense fear or discomfort. During these attacks there is an abrupt onset of multiple symptoms of autonomic arousal such as:

- palpitations;
- tachycardia;
- trembling;
- dyspnoea;
- choking;
- sweating;
- chest pain;
- nausea;
- dizziness;
- paraesthesias;
- chills;
- hot flushes; and
- feelings of impending doom, for example fear of losing control or dying.

Many patients with panic attacks begin to anticipate further panic attacks, and as a result of this anxiety, start avoiding situations where a panic attack might occur (for example, agoraphobia or fear of open places).

Panic disorder often presents to the primary care practitioner or nurse with symptoms that mimic a medical disorder. For example, a patient who is having a panic attack may appear to be having a heart attack. Patients may also present once a sequel, such as occupational impairment, or secondary depression develops.

Panic disorder may involve specific brain regions including:

- the brainstem, where neurotransmitter centres may mediate the autonomic discharge seen during the panic attacks;
- the limbic system, where GABA-ergic neurones may be involved in symptoms of anticipatory anxiety; and
- the frontal cortex, which may be responsible for mediating avoidance behaviours performed to prevent further panic attacks.

Patients with panic disorder may have experienced separation anxiety during childhood. There is also some evidence linking the onset of panic attacks with recent separations.

- *Medical causes:* These should be ruled out. Perhaps the most important of these is hyperthyroidism. Certain substances such as marijuana or amphetamines may precipitate panic attacks. Excessive caffeine may be a contributory factor.
- *Medication:* This is often useful in decreasing panic attacks. These respond to both tricyclic antidepressants (TCAs) and selective serotonin re-uptake inhibitors (SSRIs). Panic disorder patients are very sensitive to side-effects, so that very low doses should be used at first (for example imipramine 10 mg, fluoxetine 5 mg).
- *Psychoeducation:* Combined with reassurance this may be helpful to patients with anticipatory anxiety. In some cases, high potency benzodiazepines (for example alprazolam, clonazepam) can also be useful. However, the side-effects of dependency should always be kept in mind.
- *Cognitive-behavioural therapy:* This may also be useful in changing avoidance behaviours. Patients should be encouraged to face their fears – anxiety is not immediately dangerous, it can be diminished by relaxation, and it ultimately decreases after sufficient exposure to the feared situation.

Obsessive-compulsive disorder (OCD)

Obsessions are recurrent intrusive thoughts that the person typically experiences as senseless (for example, the idea of stabbing a loved one, or the idea that one is contaminated by germs). Compulsions are repetitive ritualized mental acts, or forms of behaviour, typically performed in response to such obsessions (for example, checking that the knives are hidden, or washing repeatedly to cleanse oneself). Common symptoms of OCD patients include cleaning, checking, counting, and hoarding.

OCD is thought to involve an overactive circuit between the pre-frontal cortex and the basal ganglia: for example, OCD is seen in patients with basal ganglia disorders (Tourette's syndrome, Sydenham's chorea) and patients with

OCD may also have motor tics. The serotonin system is important in mediating these circuits.

Onset of OCD is often in childhood. Women can sometimes also present during or after pregnancy. Patients may present to a primary practitioner or nurse with dermatitis from hand-washing, or with symptoms seen in several so-called OCD spectrum disorders such as hypochondriacal concerns in hypochondriasis, complaints of imagined ugliness in body dysmorphic disorder, and bald patches in trichotillomania or hair-pulling. Very often, though, patients are embarrassed about symptoms, and do not reveal them unless directly questioned.

Serotonin re-uptake inhibitors (clomipramine or the SSRIs) are the medications of choice. These may have to be used in relatively high doses (for example fluoxetine 60 mg). Response to medication is often slow, so that a reasonable trial is 10 to 12 weeks of medication.

In addition, cognitive-behavioural treatments can be useful. People with OCD should be encouraged to gradually expose themselves to increased numbers of feared stimuli without reacting compulsively (for example, touching a dirty surface and not washing). The family should be encouraged to help with this exposure. Patients and their families can be informed that such exposure actually results in reduction of the overactive brain circuits in OCD.

Psychoeducation is essential, and referral to a patient support group may be useful.

Social phobia

Social phobia is characterized by marked and persistent fear of specific social situations (for example, talking, eating, or writing in public). The individual believes that he or she will be either embarrassed or humiliated. When exposed to the relevant social situation, the patient will blush and demonstrate other physical symptoms of anxiety. In generalized social phobia there is fear of most social situations, while in limited social phobia symptoms are more restricted.

Social phobia typically presents to the primary care practitioner or nurse because of complications such as substance abuse or secondary depression. Information on the neurobiology of social phobia is relatively limited. It is a known fact that mercury poisoning sometimes results in increased shyness and timidity.

Cognitive-behavioural therapy is particularly important in social phobia. Again, this involves facing the fear, with gradual desensitization to the social situation, and reframing cognitions about this situation.

Generalized social phobia does not typically respond well to tricyclic antidepressants. The SSRIs may be more useful. In addition, monoamine oxidase inhibitors (MAOIs) have been very helpful, although this may mean having to follow dietary restrictions.

Beta-blockers given just prior to the feared social situation are often useful for limited social phobia. Psychoeducation is essential, and referral to a patient support group may be useful.

Specific phobia

A specific phobia is characterized by a marked and persistent fear, cued by the presence or anticipation of a specific object or situation (for example animals, heights, seeing blood, or flying). Exposure to the cue typically provokes an immediate anxiety response, often leading to avoidance behaviour. Although specific phobia is very common it does not typically result in presentation to a primary practitioner for treatment. Treatment is usually behavioural.

Post-traumatic stress disorder (PTSD)

Post-traumatic stress disorder occurs after exposure to a very serious traumatic event such as combat or rape. Several symptom clusters are seen:

- the traumatic event is persistently re-experienced (for instance recurrent and distressing recollections, dreams, re-enactments);

- there is persistent avoidance of stimuli associated with the trauma and numbing of general responsiveness (for instance avoidance of thoughts, feelings, or conversations associated with the trauma, inability to recall an important aspect of the trauma, and restricted range of affect): and
- there are persistent symptoms of arousal (for example insomnia, irritability, difficulty in concentrating, and hypervigilance).

Where symptoms persist for less than four weeks, a diagnosis of acute stress disorder may be made.

Patients may present to primary care practitioners or nurse with sequelae such as substance abuse or secondary depression.

Psychotherapy is often useful. This typically comprises working through the trauma by talking about the events and expressing emotions within a supportive relationship. Psychoeducation is essential, and referral to a patient support group may be useful.

Medication is usually directed at particular symptom clusters. In particular, antidepressants may be helpful in increasing mood stability and decreasing anxiety in these patients.

Prevention of PTSD may also be an important part of the primary care practitioner's or nurse's intervention. For example, the nurse may encourage debriefing sessions after the occurrence of stressful events in the community.

Generalized anxiety disorder

Generalized anxiety disorder is characterized by excessive anxiety and worry, on more days than not for at least six months, about a number of events or activities such as work or school performance. The patient finds it difficult to control the worry, and the worry is associated with somatic symptoms (for instance restlessness, being easily fatigued, difficulty in concentrating, and irritability).

Generalized anxiety disorder should be differentiated from an adjustment disorder with anxiety. This occurs in response to an identifiable stressor, and does not persist once the stressor has terminated.

Patients may present to the primary care practitioner or nurse with a variety of somatic symptoms, or with co-morbid depressive symptoms.

Both generalized anxiety disorder and adjustment disorder with anxiety may respond to reassurance or supportive psychotherapy. However, if the patient needs long-term medication then consider buspirone or antidepressants. These can be extremely helpful in the treatment of generalized anxiety disorder.

Nursing management for anxiety disorders

Counselling the patient and the family

- Educate the patient and the family to recognize the signs and symptoms of anxiety early to prevent escalation of symptoms and loss of control.
- Approach the patient calmly and assist the patient to label the anxiety.
- Encourage the patient to practise *relaxation methods* (such as slow, relaxed breathing) to reduce physical symptoms of anxiety.
- Identify exaggerated fears, which occur with anxiety (for example, patient feels a pounding heart and fears he or she is having a heart attack).
- Discuss ways to challenge these fears when they occur (for example, patient reminds him or herself: 'I am not having a heart attack. This is a panic attack, and it will pass in a few minutes.').

In the case of phobias, i.e. anxiety related to specific situations, plan a series of steps to enable the patient to confront and get used to a feared situation.

For example:
- Identify a small first step towards facing the feared situation (for example, take a short walk away from home with a family member).

- Help the patient to practise this step repeatedly until it is no longer frightening.
- Don't let the patient leave the feared situation if it still causes anxiety, until the fear subsides (this will always occur after a few minutes).
- Move the patient on to a slightly more difficult step and repeat the procedure (for example, spending a longer period away from home).
- Do not let the patient use alcohol or drugs to help cope with feared situations.
- Identify the patient's current life problems or social stressors. Focus on small, specific steps patients might take towards managing these problems.
- Encourage patients to take regular exercise.
- Support the patient to build on previously successful coping methods, and discuss alternative methods of dealing with the anxiety that fit into the patient's situation.
- Help the patient to identify support systems.
- Inform and educate the patient of the importance of abstaining from caffeine, nicotine, and any other central nervous system stimulants.

Note: Screening for the presence of anxiety disorders should be part of the general primary care evaluation. If anxiety is present, patients should not simply be labelled as 'anxious' or 'neurotic' but should preferably be diagnosed specifically.

This in turn allows the primary care practitioner and nurse to plan a specific treatment strategy. The prognosis for anxiety disorders can be very favourable, so non-responsive patients should be referred for further evaluation and treatment.

15 Somatoform disorders

This chapter covers a difficult group of disorders that are common in the primary health care situation. Nurses are advised to consult a more comprehensive text for amplification.

Somatoform disorders

The somatoform disorders are a group of disorders that have physical symptoms, for example nausea, dizziness, and pain, for which no adequate medical explanation can be found. The symptoms are serious enough to impair the patient's social or occupational functioning. There may be positive evidence, or strong presumption, that the symptoms are linked to psychological factors or conflicts. The symptom production is not intentional so the patient does not experience a sense of controlling this in any way. There is no demonstrable organic lesion. This is a worrying group of disorders because vague symptoms may be the early presentation of some medical conditions. Consultation in these cases is important.

Many of these syndromes are closely related and it seems likely that common aetiological processes are involved. Authorities differ as to how these disorders should be classified.

DSM-IV describes five types of somatoform disorder, namely:

- somatization disorder;
- conversion disorder;

- hypochondriasis;
- body dysmorphic disorder; and
- pain disorder.

Somatization disorder (hysteria/Briquet's syndrome)

Essential diagnostic features

This type of disorder is characterized by:
- a variety of physical complaints affecting various organs;
- onset before the age of thirty;
- recurrent and multiple complaints of several years' duration;
- significant functional impairment;
- the fact that medical and/or surgical treatment has been sought;
- symptoms that are neither due to a medical disorder nor intentionally produced;
- symptoms that include gastro-intestinal, sexual, and pseudoneurological pain.

Epidemiology

Onset usually occurs before the age of thirty with a chronic but fluctuating course. The disorder occurs in 5 to 10 per cent of the primary care population. The ratio of female to male patients is 20 to 1.

Clinical presentation

Complaints are often presented in a dramatic way, or are part of a complicated medical history in which many physical diagnoses have been considered. It is often difficult to get a clear history of onset, or of why the patient has come for help. Patients are unusually invested in their illness and recount names and medical events in great detail.

Histories given to different physicians tend to show inconsistencies and these patients often receive medical care from a number of physicians, sometimes simultaneously.

They tend to be extensively investigated and over-treated medically and surgically – they eventually undergo three times as many surgical operations as either sick or healthy controls. It is often extremely difficult to decide whether the behaviour of these patients is under unconscious control or whether they are malingering. For full diagnostic criteria a textbook should be consulted.

Co-existing disorders

- anxiety;
- depressed mood; or
- histrionic and anti-social personality disorder.

Differential diagnosis

- major depression;
- schizophrenia; or
- medical illness.

Treatment

A specialist opinion is probably necessary to satisfy the patient. Thereafter somatization disorder patients need a long-term empathic relationship with a single physician (or nurse in underserved areas), who needs to build up trust to hold the patient. Patients are helped to cope with their symptoms and stop 'doctor shopping'. Medication should be used with caution. Somatization patients tend to use medication erratically and unreliably. Antidepressants or anxiolytics may be effective but there is a risk of psychoactive substance-induced psychotic disorder.

Conversion disorder (or hysterical neurosis, conversion type)

Essential diagnostic features

These include:

- alteration or loss of voluntary motor function or sensation;
- no known neurological condition;
- association between the symptoms or signs and psychological factors that are not intentionally produced (as in malingering or factitious disorder); and
- specified types: motor or sensory system deficit, seizures, or mixed picture.

The syndrome should not be diagnosed solely because an organic cause for the physical symptoms cannot be found. Follow-up studies have shown high rates (60 per cent) of overt organic disease having developed within a few years in patients previously diagnosed as having conversion symptoms.

Epidemiology

Conversion disorders are more common among rural and less-educated people and in some high-stress situations such as combat. The condition is more common in women.

Aetiology

Conversion disorders are thought to be an expression of a psychological conflict or need. The symptoms are not intentionally produced and cannot be explained by any physical disorder or known pathophysiologic mechanism.

Clinical features

The most common are neurological symptoms such as paralysis, aphonia, seizures, co-ordination disturbances, blindness, anosmia, and paraesthesia. Often the symptoms and signs do not fit into recognized anatomical or pathological patterns. The course of a conversion disorder is most often of short duration with sudden onset, often in clear reaction to stress. A conversion symptom is likely to involve a single symptom during a given episode, but may vary in site and nature with subsequent episodes (so-called symptom substitution). Increased anxiety levels may be present. An attitude of lack of concern (la belle indifference) is sometimes present but has little diagnostic value.

Associated features

In 'primary gain' the patient retains an internal conflict or need out of awareness (for example, after an argument the patient loses his or her voice [aphonia]). In 'secondary gain' the patient avoids a particularly noxious activity: for example, with a 'paralyzed' hand a soldier can avoid firing a gun.

Differential diagnosis

- Major depression and/or medical condition.

Treatment

Resolution is usually spontaneous but the clinician should appreciate the emotional stress represented by the symptom and take it seriously. Simplistic or degrading magical solutions such as placebo injections are not appropriate. The patient needs reassurance. Stress factors must be explored at the time of treating the symptoms with appropriate physical non-invasive therapy such as speech therapy or practice for aphonia, or physiotherapy for paralysis.

Patients often benefit from culturally congruent interventions and should not be discouraged from consulting spiritual healers. Anxiolytics or antidepressants may be effective in some cases.

Course and prognosis

The longer such patients have been in the sick role (especially patients with dependent personality traits) the more difficult the treatment will be.

Hypochondriasis

Essential diagnostic features

The patient may worry excessively about having a serious disease based on his or her personal misinterpretation of physical symptoms, despite appropriate medical evaluation and reassurance. The condition is not delusional; there is impairment of ability to function in their personal, social, and occupational roles; the duration is longer than six months and it is not due to anxiety disorder, obsessive-compulsive disorder, major depression, or any other somatoform disorder.

Epidemiology

The condition is equally common in males and females. It occurs in 1 per cent of psychiatric patients, with a peak incidence between the ages of thirty and forty.

Aetiology

Theories include:

- misinterpretation of body sensations;
- a learnt sick role;
- a variant of some other mental disorder;
- psychodynamic theory; and
- hostile wishes transferred into symptoms.

Clinical features

The patient has an exaggerated preoccupation with bodily functions such as heartbeat, sweating, or minor physical abnormalities (occasional cough). The feared disease may involve several systems at different times or simultaneously. There may also be a preoccupation with a specific organ (cardiac neurosis). The most common regions of the body involved are head and neck, and abdomen and chest, in that order. The bodily systems most affected are musculoskeletal, gastro-intestinal, and the central nervous system. Complaints are often vague and dramatic and vary with life stresses.

The disorder can begin at any age, and it usually has a chronic course. There is often some impairment in social or occupational functioning due to the patient's constant preoccupation with his or her health. Complications are often secondary to efforts to obtain medical care (a risk of multiple diagnostic procedures). Doctor-shopping and deterioration in the 'doctor-patient' relationship with frustration and anger on both sides are common. This disorder is frequently seen in general practice. Patients usually feel offended at the suggestion that their fears are unwarranted and often refuse referral for mental health care. Anxiety, depressed mood, and obsessive-compulsive personality traits are often observed.

Differential diagnosis

- Medical disorders such as multiple sclerosis, Aids, and systemic lupus erythematosus.
- Schizophrenia or major depression, in which the belief that, in reality, one has an undiagnosed or serious illness reaches delusional intensity. In schizophrenia the ideas tend to be most bizarre.

- Somatization disorder.
- Anxiety states and panic disorder.

Treatment

- Schedule regular supportive listening, cognitive psychotherapy, or group therapy (the patient is taken seriously).
- Schedule regular physical examinations.
- Specifically treat any psychiatric disorder. Monosymptomatic hypochondriasis of delusional proportions may respond to treatment with pimozide.

The course and prognosis is fair to good with understanding management.

Nursing management

Essential information for patient and family

- Stress often produces physical symptoms.
- The focus should be on managing the symptoms, not on discovering the cause.
- Cure may not be possible, the goal should be to live the best life possible even if symptoms continue.

Counselling the patient and family

- Acknowledge that the patient's physical symptoms are real. (They are not lies or inventions.)
- Reinforce improvement in the patient. Try not to reinforce symptoms.
- Ask the patient what he or she thinks is causing the symptoms. Offer appropriate reassurance (for example, abdominal pain does not indicate cancer). Advise patients not to focus on medical worries.
- Discuss emotional stressors that were present when the symptoms began.
- Suggest relaxation methods that can help relieve symptoms related to tension (headaches, neck, or back pain).

- Acute cases may need brief rest and relief from stress. After the acute period, encourage exercise and enjoyable activities. The patient need not wait until all symptoms are gone before returning to normal routines.
- Schedule appointments for patients with more chronic complaints. Regular time-limited appointments with the same doctor may prevent more frequent, urgent visits.

Medication prescribed by medical practitioner

- Avoid unnecessary diagnostic testing or prescription of new medication for each new symptom.
- Antidepressant medication (e.g. imipramine 25–75 mg a day) may be helpful in some cases (for example, headache, irritable bowel syndrome, or atypical chest pain).
- Avoid repeated referrals to specialists. Patients are best managed by one primary health care physician or nurse. Patients may be offended by psychiatric referral and seek additional medical consultation elsewhere.

16 Sleep disorders

The significance of poor sleep and resultant daytime problems with sleepiness may seem trivial to some. One night of bad sleep can easily be compensated for the next night, but years of poor sleep can have significant consequences. Sleepiness during the day, whether caused by insomnia or hypersomnia, has been shown to increase the accident rate by up to five times and underlying depression and anxiety is exacerbated. There are three groups of sleep disorders, namely:

- true insomnia;
- hypersomnia; and
- parasomnias.

It is initially important to determine whether or not a specific individual's sleep characteristics are abnormal and are not a normal variant. Natural short sleepers can sleep for as little as four hours a night and natural long sleepers for ten. The elderly also experience a dramatic decrease in total sleeping hours in addition to reduced quality and more awakenings during the night. If this pattern is not accompanied by daytime fatigue it can be normal.

True insomnia

This is defined as the inability to get sufficient sleep at night with resulting deficits in function the following day. The commonest causes and treatments follow.

Depression

The patient is able to fall asleep easily but awakens in the early morning and is unable to get back to sleep. This pattern is usually associated with other daytime features of depression.

Treatment

Treatment is as for depression. For severe insomnia more sedative night-time tricyclic antidepressants may sometimes be indicated.

Restless legs syndrome (RLS) and periodic limb movement disorder (PLMD)

This is a common condition found in 5 per cent of the population. RLS causes an unpleasant sensation in the lower legs or arms, which produces an overwhelming desire to move the legs. The sensations differ among patients and occur at any time of day when the legs are still. These symptoms are particularly severe at night. Most patients with RLS, and some without, have PLMD once they have fallen asleep. PLMD is characterized by a rhythmical twitch in the lower limb muscles that causes fragmentation of sleep.

Treatment

Prescribe clonazepam (Rivotril), commencing with a dosage of 0,5 mg at night. The dosage can be increased to 2–3 mg per night. If this is unsuccessful, carbidopa (Sinemet 25/100) can be tried, dose half to two tablets at night.

Psychophysiological insomnia

Patients typically feel very tired at bedtime but once they are in bed with the light off they find that they are wide awake. They then become very anxious and frustrated, and a state of conditioned arousal occurs. They complain of their minds racing. Physiological parameters such as pulse rate and muscle tone increase and this further prevents sleep onset.

Treatment

Institute general sleep improvement measures. Medication can be used as an adjunct when necessary, for example every third night. The general sleep improvement measures are sleep restriction, sleep hygiene, and writing up a sleep diary (see 'Nursing management' p. 176). Ongoing help and objective assessment is often necessary for up to eight weeks for complete resolution. The sleep time is gradually increased to the normal amount as the quality of sleep improves. A centre for sleep disorders should be contacted in cases of resistant insomnia or suspicion of PLMD.

Hypersomnia

Hypersomnia presents as excessive daytime sleepiness despite an adequate amount of sleep at night. Sleepiness may occur while watching television, reading, working, during lectures, or even while driving a car.

Narcolepsy

The condition usually starts in young adulthood and has a familial trend. Symptoms include:
- chronic fatigue;
- sleep attacks during the day;
- cataplexy, which is a sudden onset of paralysis of either the whole body or part of it with emotion – for instance laughter or anger;
- hallucinations at the onset of sleep or on waking; and
- sleep paralysis, which is total body paralysis for a few minutes after waking.

Diagnosis can be confirmed at a centre for sleep disorders by means of a MSLT (Multiple Sleep Latency Test) and an overnight polysomnogram.

Treatment

Stimulants, including pemoline (Dynalert) and methylphenidate (Ritalin) are prescribed for sleepiness. Clomipramine (Anafranil) can be prescribed for cataplexy.

Obstructive sleep apnoea

This condition is common (10 per cent) in males between the ages of forty and sixty. Symptoms include:

- *during the night* there is severe snoring, 'holding of breath', restlessness and sweating, and the patient wakes up choking;
- *upon waking* the patient feels tired and has a dry mouth, headache, or hangover feeling; and
- *during the day* there is mild to severe sleepiness as above, and personality change.

Examination may reveal a long palate with a swollen uvula.

Diagnosis can be confirmed at a centre for sleep disorders where overnight monitoring of respiratory parameters can be done.

Treatment

If the condition is mild, weight loss, conservative treatment to the nose (for instance treat rhinitis), ENT surgery including nose and/or palate, and an orthodontic device should be considered. If the condition is moderate to severe, a nasal continuous positive airways pressure (CPAP) device is indicated.

Parasomnias

Parasomnias are strange happenings during sleep. The condition is usually benign, particularly in children, and they grow out of it on reaching puberty. Parasomnias only need to be treated if they are very disruptive and particularly if they have not resolved by puberty. Differential diagnosis: nocturnal epilepsy.

Sleepwalking

The patient gets up and walks around the house, usually within the first three hours of sleep. A familial history of sleepwalking is common.

Night terrors

Within the first three hours of sleep, the child sits up and screams. Parents are unable to either comfort or wake the child. This lasts for ten to fifteen minutes, after which the child sleeps normally. (Nightmares usually occur in the latter part of the night and the child is easily consoled.)

Nursing management

Essential information for patient and family

- Temporary sleep problems are common at times of stress or physical illness.
- The normal amount of sleep varies widely and usually decreases with age.

Counselling of patient and family

Help clients to maintain a regular sleep routine by teaching them about sleep restriction, sleep hygiene, and by encouraging them to keep a sleep diary.

- *Sleep restriction* involves allowing the patient to spend the number of hours currently being slept, in bed. In other words, a patient who sleeps for only four hours should go to bed at midnight and rise at 04:00.
- *Sleep hygiene* involves taking the following steps. Patients should:
  - not consume caffeine after lunchtime;
  - reduce alcohol and nicotine consumption;
  - take regular exercise during the day;
  - spend only fifteen minutes trying to fall asleep and if this proves to be unsuccessful get out of bed and keep busy, for example by reading a book or watching television until the onset of sleepiness, and then go back to bed and try again;

- rise at a set time every morning; and
- not nap during the day.
- Writing up a *sleep diary* involves recording significant features such as the time slept and the number of awakenings during the night.

These measures seem extreme at first but they usually bring about significant changes in sleep within a week

Medication prescribed by a medical practitioner.

- Treat underlying psychiatric or physical condition.
- Make changes to medication, as appropriate.
- Hypnotic medication may be used intermittently (e.g. benzodiazepines such as oxazepam 15–30 mg at bedtime). Risk of dependence increases significantly after fourteen days of use. Avoid hypnotic medication in cases of chronic insomnia.

Note that there is no specific medication that will cure fatigue. If the fatigue results *from* a physical or mental problem, medication for these problems may reduce some of the underlying fatigue. Sometimes certain antidepressants are useful for some people.

Medications that claim to lessen fatigue can lead to addiction. Patients have to use increasing doses of the drug and symptoms become much worse when they discontinue the medication. These medications are also harmful if taken during pregnancy or if used with alcohol and other drugs.

17 Difficult patients: personality disorders

Difficult patients that may present in a PHC setting include those with:
- personality disorders; and
- aggressive patients.

Personality disorders

Personality is an enduring style of behaviour that is unique to each individual. It influences a person's interpersonal relationships and reactions to events. The characteristic behaviours that comprise personality are referred to as personality traits. A personality disorder occurs when the traits are maladaptive, inflexible, have persisted through life, and result in impairment in function of the individual or in marked interpersonal problems.

Epidemiology

Personality disorder is thought to be present in 10 to 20 per cent of the general population. The prevalence figures are much higher in a psychiatric population. Age of onset is in adolescence, but a personality disorder cannot be diagnosed until the patient is over eighteen years of age. Late onset usually has another cause, which must be looked into. The intensity of symptoms of some personality disorders seems to diminish with age. They may however become exaggerated in a patient with dementia.

Aetiology

Biological theories include genetic factors, electrophysiological abnormalities such as abnormal electroencephalograms in antisocial personality, and neurohormonal and neurotransmitter abnormalities.

Many psychosocial theories exist (refer to standard textbooks).

Classification

Table 17.1 shows how the *Diagnostic and statistical manual of mental disorders*, 4th edition (DSM-IV), classifies personality disorders into various clusters and subtypes.

Table 17.1 DSM-IV personality disorders

Cluster A
Paranoid personality disorder
Schizoid personality disorder
Schizotypal personality disorder

Cluster B
Antisocial personality disorder
Borderline personality disorder
Histrionic personality disorder
Narcissistic personality disorder

Cluster C
Avoidant personality disorder
Dependent personality disorder
Obsessive-compulsive personality disorder

Cluster A

Paranoid personality disorder

These individuals are mistrustful and suspicious. They tend to be cold, aloof, and hostile. Their patterns of thinking are rigid and they have difficulty in dealing with criticism.

Schizoid personality disorder

These individuals keep to themselves, prefer their own company, and pursue solitary activities.

Schizotypal personality disorder

People with schizotypal personality disorder are characteristically isolated and aloof. Odd behaviour and thinking patterns may be displayed, namely magical thinking, eccentricity, strange speech, and limited emotional responses (blunted affect).

As a group, Cluster A personality disorder individuals rarely present voluntarily for treatment. In times of crisis they have a tendency to develop psychotic illnesses.

Cluster B

Antisocial personality disorder

A history of conduct disorder stemming from childhood and adolescence is usual, i.e. lying, stealing, truancy, and fighting. The hallmark of this disorder is callous behaviour with lack of remorse. Behaviours include deceitfulness, irresponsibility, aggressiveness, inability or lack of interest in holding down a job, and a history of arrests for criminal activity. They freely attribute blame to others.

Borderline personality disorder (BPD)

This disorder is marked by instability in interpersonal relationships. Emotions are manifested by intense anger, an intolerance of being alone, mood fluctuations, and irritability. Lifestyles are characterized by living from one crisis to the next.

During periods of crisis, self-destructive behaviour is often exhibited in the form of self-mutilation and multiple suicide attempts. There may be a history of early childhood abuse.

Histrionic personality disorder

These individuals are superficially charming, but their emotions are shallow and volatile. They are overly dramatic, attention seeking, and suggestible. Their interactions with others are often characterized by inappropriately seductive or provocative behaviour.

Narcissistic personality disorder

An inflated self-esteem and a sense of self-importance predominate. These persons view the world as revolving around themselves. They are preoccupied with 'self' issues, namely success, power, and beauty. They want to be considered special. They crave admiration and have a sense of entitlement. Interpersonal relationships are characterized by exploitation and lack of empathy for the feelings of others.

Cluster B personality-disordered patients frequently experience brief episodes of depression. Under certain circumstances they may have brief psychotic episodes. Manipulation of loved ones, friends, and even the health worker is common behaviour.

Cluster C

Avoidant personality disorder

These individuals are shy, introverted, and lack self-esteem. They fear rejection and embarrassment and therefore avoid situations or interpersonal contact that may result in these situations. Social activity therefore remains minimal despite their desire for it.

Dependent personality disorder

Submissiveness and self-doubt lead to clinging behaviours and fears of separation from those they rely on. They are unable to make decisions without advice and reassurance from others. There is difficulty in assuming responsibility for major areas of their lives. They constantly seek approval and are even afraid to take care of themselves.

Obsessive-compulsive personality disorder

These individuals are perfectionistic and inflexible. They are preoccupied with minor details and are very demanding in what they expect from others. They are overly conscientious about their work and rarely delegate for fear that others will not meet their high standards.

Management

The nurse often has to treat co-morbid psychiatric disorders or specific emotional problems and crises. An underlying personality disorder makes the co-morbid psychiatric or medical disorder more difficult to treat and usually worsens the prognosis of the psychiatric or medical disorder. Nurses should not make the error of neglecting treatment of the psychiatric disorder while labelling the patient as simply having a personality disorder.

Personality also influences the way in which patients present with medical or physical disorders. A nurse who understands this concept will experience improved medical diagnostic skills and patient compliance. A healthier and more understanding relationship with the patient will also ensue.

The treatment of the different personality disorders usually involves specific forms of psychotherapy conducted by a skilled therapist. Some patients, of necessity, remain in psychotherapy for years, while others undergo psychotherapy intermittently when the need arises. Except sometimes in the case of BPD, medication is not generally used to treat personality disorders but may be used in the treatment of co-morbid psychiatric disorders.

Nurses need to be familiar with the management of the problems that are peculiar to personality disorder patients.

Manipulation

While overt forms of manipulation are easily recognized, the more subtle forms often go unheeded until the nurse is overwhelmed by the patient's manoeuvres. Obtaining collateral information to verify patient symptoms or complaints is essential. Relatives who have been the victims of manipulation need to be taught how to handle the patient. The nurse needs to confront the patient in a non-judgemental manner without feeling guilty.

Seduction

This can vary from simple flattery to overt attempts at sexual seduction. The nurse should always be alert to this possibility with patients. Often the patient's goal is to feel special and treatment should address this.

Demands

These may take various forms such as numerous calls for help at odd times, demands for medication, insistence that the nurse should reprimand relatives, or repeated requests for time off from work. The nurse should set firm limits for the patient, but the patient should know that the nurse is still available when genuinely needed.

Low self-esteem

Patients need to recognize that the problem is usually their own faulty perception of themselves. The nurse needs to restructure the thinking patterns of these patients, and encourage them to concentrate on positive aspects of themselves. Where available, local assertiveness training courses or social skills groups should be utilized.

Dependency on the nurse

Both the nurse and the patient need to realize that this behaviour is unhealthy. The nurse must overcome any feelings of gratification that this type of patient provides. The nurse should set firm limits on the number of visits, the timing of visits, and the type of requests for help.

The diagnosis of personality disorder is made only after other possibilities have been excluded. The label is not applied lightly. When in doubt, consultation is essential. These patients can be extremely difficult and take up precious time and resources. If health workers do not have a good understanding of these individuals, they can cause bitter divisions among staff.

Nursing management

It is important for the nurse to realize that people who suffer from personality disorders demonstrate a repetitive pattern of behaviour that manifests specific deficits within the personality structure – they experience problems in *living*, rather than specific symptoms as with other psychiatric disorders. It is maladjusted *behaviour* patterns that indicate pathology that is outwardly directed towards and against others.

It seems as though this stems from faulty emotional and moral development during the first three years of life. The primary nursing care goal for patients experiencing behavioural disruptions is to bring about changes in behaviour resulting in healthier functioning.

The PHC nurse could apply the following principles in managing personality disorders:

- Educate the patient to manage stressful life situations, as these increase aberrant behaviour.
- Symptoms are usually a mask for feelings of inadequacy, worthlessness, and fear. The nurse can use empathy, unconditional acceptance, and interpersonal skills to reflect and help the patient understand and manage this in an appropriate way.
- Set limits and structure the environment to decrease manipulative, aggressive, and impulsive behaviour as these are unhealthy ways of coping.
- Set limits according to the patient's ability to accept responsibility for himself or herself.
- Always be direct, honest, and consistent in your approach to the patient to enforce positive behaviour.
- Confront maladaptive behaviour and explore alternative, adaptive strategies.

These patients seldom see themselves as in need of help. They are 'actors' attempting to fool others, but ultimately they deprive themselves of meaningful and satisfying relationships. Often they do not even realize what they are missing.

Aggressive behaviour

In a primary health care setting, the nurse often encounters patients who are threatening, aggressive, and violent. It is therefore important that she or he can understand the dynamics behind this behaviour, and manage it appropriately.

Aggressive patients are not only seen in psychiatric settings. They may be encountered at all levels of primary or secondary medical care.

Causes of aggressive behaviour

Substance abuse (alcohol or drugs)

The use of these substances frequently causes disinhibited behaviour. Aggression can occur either during usage or upon withdrawal.

Bipolar mood disorder

The manic phase of this illness may cause the patient to be extremely euphoric or irritable and aggressive.

Schizophrenia

Certain types of this disorder (for example, paranoid sub-types) can result in suspicion and aggression.

Epilepsy

In some individuals this disorder may present with violent and aggressive behaviour. This type of epilepsy is sometimes referred to as a psychomotor seizure.

Mentally-challenged individuals

These patients lack the ability to respond appropriately to social situations and can easily become aggressive. They may also be subject to abuse by others and this may make them violent.

Head injuries

People who have sustained severe head injuries sometimes undergo personality changes. They can become easily irritated and aggressive. Forms of epilepsy may aggravate this.

Dementia

Patients with dementia, particularly the aged, can become paranoid and aggressive.

Brief history

A brief history from a relative or friend can give some clues to the cause of the aggressive behaviour.

Rate of onset

Sudden onset may indicate substance abuse or epilepsy. A shorter period of onset, for example one to two weeks, could point to a mood disorder. A relatively protracted period of illness is compatible with schizophrenia or dementia.

Precipitating factors

The presence of a recent psychosocial stressor is important in the development of mental illness (particularly bipolar mood disorder). Aggressive episodes may be caused by substance abuse or sudden cessation of psychotropic medication.

Presence and type of hallucinations

Auditory hallucinations are more common in schizophrenia, while visual hallucinations are usually common in substance abusers. Epileptic patients experience a wide range of perceptual distortions, for example illusions, hallucinations, and other strange phenomena.

Maladjustment

A history of lifelong maladjustment to society may suggest that an individual is mentally challenged or has some type of personality disorder.

Medical management

Control with medication

- Clothiapine (Etomine) 40–80 mg intramuscularly or intravenously. Repeat when necessary to a maximum dosage of 240 mg/24 hours (in an 80 kg adult); or
- Haloperidol 5–10 mg intramuscularly 2-hourly if necessary. Do not exceed 60 mg in 24 hours; or
- Diazepam 10 mg administered intravenously, slowly in epileptic patients. Other drugs may cause or worsen seizures (diazepam may be added to clothiapine or haloperidol for additional sedation); or
- Chlorpromazine 50–100 mg by mouth. Avoid administering this drug intramuscularly or intravenously.

In all the above cases try to get a blood pressure reading and pulse rate before administering any drugs.

Other useful drugs include zuclopenthixol acetate (Clopixol Acuphase, which lasts three days), clonazepam and lorazepam.

Remember that the above doses are only guidelines. In some cases patients may only respond to higher or lower doses. Monitor sedated patients carefully. At a later stage, once the patient is controlled, perform a careful physical and mental state examination to make a diagnosis.

Nursing mangement guidelines

Remember that an aggressive patient is in distress, but can also be dangerous. Take the following measures:

- Be prepared! Be very clear on management before anything happens.
- Build trust by being open and honest; make suggestions rather than giving commands. Invite participation from the patient and redirect action.
- Get help, exercise caution, allow for escape, and identify yourself.
- Try to calm the patient, speak gently. ('I can see that you are very upset.') Avoid any sudden or threatening action.
- Listen to the patient – alone if it is safe.
- Do not loosen any bonds. Maintain some distance between yourself and the patient.
- Set limits and control by providing clear, concise explanations for expectations, rules, and regulations.
- Listen to the patient's complaints and attempt to identify their legitimacy.
- Show unconditional acceptance by allowing the patient to express his or her feelings of anger, resentment, and bitterness, regardless of behaviour.
- Together with the patient, identify the cause of the aggressive behaviour and negotiate methods of management to assist in the development of socially acceptable patterns of behaviour.
- Educate the family on how to channel aggressive behaviour into other constructive and socially acceptable activities.

- Protect and control the patient's behaviour through external controls, e.g. 'If you do not stop banging the table, you will go back to your room'(consequences of behaviour).
- Do not contradict or argue with the patient.
- Do not make false promises.
- Attempt to negotiate treatment ('Medication to calm you.')
- Try to persuade the patient to surrender any weapon in his or her possession.
- Do not attempt any heroics.
- If the patient has to be restrained ensure that you have enough help to control each limb without hurting the patient. Covering the patient with a mattress or blanket is useful. Approach from behind.

Once the patient has been sedated and/or restrained:
- Do not leave the patient alone – a staff member or relative should stay to explain reassuringly what has been done and why. This needs to be done several times.
- Remove any dangerous weapons, objects, or drugs from the patient.
- Reassess every fifteen minutes. Check:
  - vital signs, BP, pulse, respiration;
  - limbs, if restrained, for compression or ischaemia;
  - level of consciousness; and
  - mental state – the person should be calm on approach; if still struggling or aggressive, they may need more sedation.
- Transfer as soon as possible to your referral hospital for full evaluation and management. The patient must be escorted, and observations and treatment continued on the trip.

18 Ageing, mental illness, and community care

Ageing is the progressive decline in function and performance that accompanies advancing years. It is multifactorial in aetiology, partly inborn (primary ageing) and partly environmental (secondary ageing) due to wearing out by 'accumulated stress and strain'. The effects of ageing and hence the experience of ageing and its social consequences may be discussed under the headings as set out below.

Demographic effects

Population trends demonstrate a rising percentage of individuals aged sixty-five and over. Currently the proportion of elderly in the more developed countries is approximately 15 per cent as opposed to 4 per cent in the less developed countries. But it is estimated that the proportion of elderly in Africa will double within the next seventeen years. In general, this increase is due less to any marked improvement in life expectancy, than to the effect of reduced fertility rates and decreasing mortality rates in the young. Thus, future demographic trends around the world will depend on measures of population control and improved health services. While the international trend is to describe as 'elderly' persons aged sixty-five and over, less developed countries would include those over the age of sixty in order to highlight the current needs of this age group.

The increase in the numbers of people in the upper age brackets has enormous financial implications. In countries such as England, the elderly occupy 40 per cent of the out-patient and 33 per cent of the in-patient physician's time.

Approximately 30 to 40 per cent of this group is psychiatri-cally impaired while 80 per cent suffer from some physical illness, and many from both. Thus the need for setting up effective services for the elderly becomes quite clear. The most common psychiatric illness in the elderly is *depression* (see Chapter 13), at a prevalence of about 18 per cent in women and 12 per cent in men. Although *dementia* (see Chapter 19) has a prevalence rate of only 5 to 10 per cent, depending on age category, we can adequately manage and contain depression in the elderly, while in dementia this is not the case. Currently there is no cure for dementia.

Until recently, the elderly occupied up to 50 per cent of all psychiatric hospital beds, and accounted for some 20 per cent of all admissions. More recently, many of these patients have been placed in the community with an ever-increasing burden on the community, and on non-governmental organisations and individual caregivers. There is currently an international trend to sell off the large tracts of land belonging to psychiatric hospitals, and to repatriate the patients into the community. This process is affordable and benefits both parties, namely the state and the community, provided these funds are re-invested, since the community cannot carry this burden without assistance. Notwith-standing, a 'hard core' of some 15 per cent of patients (of all ages) will always require hospitalization, owing to the higher degree of medical and nursing care necessary. Hospital-ization is also necessary for the treatment and stabilization of the acutely ill elderly who cannot be managed in a com-munity setting. Regarding community care, one also has to remember that over the last fifty years the proportion of 'middle-aged' (between thirty-five and sixty-five) to elderly has dwindled from 10 : 1 to some 4 : 1 in more developed countries. Over the same period the proportion of middle-aged women (the caregivers of the elderly) going out to work has risen from some 10 to 60 per cent. Less developed countries are pursuing this trend. In less developed countries up to 50 per cent of a given population is younger than twenty-five. These in turn compete with the elderly for support from the 25- to 45- year old age group. Though the latter group has the highest income, it also has the highest HIV-infected rate. This age group is also contending with other problems of its own such as dwindling natural and economic resources, competition with the more advanced nations on an industrial and technological level, unemployment, and the effects of migration.

The resultant changes in the structural relationship between all the different age groups will greatly impinge on the community health worker.

At a more personal level, the elderly are easy victims of poor housing and poverty, pensions that cannot keep pace with the daily cost of living, and a decreasing intellect that gives rise to an inability to use financial resources to best advantage. All this requires an increase in the number of services for the elderly, namely primary health care, hospital-based services, home visiting, day hospitals, day centres, liaison services, residential and old age homes, council houses, and villages.

Physical changes

At present, in the poorer socio-economic sector of the less developed countries, the life expectancy for a female is about sixty-four and that of a male about sixty, contrasting with seventy-seven and seventy in the more affluent sector.

The causes of death in those over the age of sixty-five are generally considered to be:
- cardiovascular disease 53 per cent;
- neoplasms 17 per cent; and
- respiratory disease, 14 per cent.

There is a mutual relationship between old age and disease; disease hastens ageing and age renders the aged person more vulnerable to diseases, especially degenerative diseases.

Appearance and organ function

- Height decreases by some 8 cm by the age of eighty owing to a decrease in bone mass with an increased curvature of the spine.
- Body weight steadily decreases, while joints stiffen and osteoarthritis becomes more common.
- Skin becomes dry, thin, and wrinkled, and senile bruises appear spontaneously, most often on the forearms and legs.
- Hair becomes white and sparse.
- Deafness ensues to different degrees.
- Teeth fall out, the jaw gradually shrinks, and dentures become loose.
- Organs tend to shrink in size.
- Functional reserve, which allows adaptation to stress, declines.
- Cardiac output decreases and there is a rise in blood pressure, which, with the effects of atheroma, may lead to mycardial infarction, heart failure, or strokes.
- Lungs are more rigid, and are predisposed to chronic bronchitis and pneumonia.
- Gastro-intestinal tract diminishes in function, and this results in constipation, which is common and troublesome.
- Prostate gland englarges in males and the atrophic vagina in females may lead to urinary tract infections, which impair health and contribute to incontinence.
- Diabetes is more common together with other physical ailments to which the elderly are prone including dehydration, anaemia, cancer, and hypothermia.

Central nervous system

Mental function in the elderly is spared more than the dramatic microscopic changes in the brain would suggest. Cell loss approaches 50 per cent in some cortical areas while fewer dendritic interconnections remain between neurons. All senses decline, with deafness and failing vision leading to social isolation, while loss of the senses of smell and taste lead to a decrease in appetite.

Psychosocial effects

From the evolutionary point of view there must be some advantage for the continued survival of mankind following the end of reproductive life. Since humans are unique both in the richness and complexity of their memories and experiences and have the ability to share this knowledge with others, one presumes this to be a major reason. Unfortunately, a clear role for the elderly in a given society is yet to be defined.

Intellectual function

A small percentage of elderly persons maintain a stable IQ even at advanced ages, although the great majority demonstrate a gradual decline. Contrary to myth, memory is not dramatically affected in healthy, emotionally stable elderly people.

'Fluid intelligence' (the ability to acquire and integrate new information) is more susceptible to ageing effects than 'crystallized intelligence' (based on education and experience), which increases and offsets the former with age. Responses may be slowed but are often offset by experience and knowledge.

Sexual function

All phases of the sexual act tend to be slowed. But decreased sexual interest and activity after the age of sixty is psychological rather than physiological. Some elderly people maintain and enjoy sexual activities into the eighties, while others find intimacy, sensuality and being valued as a man or a woman sufficient.

Personality changes

Many elderly people become introverted, and as their circle of friends diminishes, so does their interest in current affairs. Soon the inner world becomes richer than the outer. Habits and routines prevail, as the difficulties in learning new ideas and skills lead to a resistance to changing beliefs and opinions. They may become preoccupied with bodily functions, especially the bowels, which could lead to hypochondriasis.

Losses experienced in old age

The hurdles that present themselves to the elderly are generally described as 'losses'. These the individual must successfully negotiate and adapt to in order to render the ageing process less stressful.

Status

Contemporary Western society is materialistic, and spiritual and traditional values count for relatively little. Despite being referred to as 'senior citizens' once their working days are over, they are seen as dependent members of society with little to offer. Early retirement can 'age' a person, and those with a high investment in a work role are at risk of losing self-esteem and becoming depressed.

Income

There is often a substantial drop in income following retirement and most people have to budget very carefully. Style of living needs to be changed and pensions that are poorly adjusted to the rate of inflation are a constant source of worry.

Health

The infirmities associated with ageing cause pain and discomfort, restrict mobility, reduce social interaction, and generally impair enjoyment of life. They also lead to increasing dependency.

Company

Retirement may place considerable strain on a marital relationship because the couple now have to live together all day.

For many, it also means loss of working colleagues and friends. Often the loss of a spouse is irreplaceable and many aged people never recover, sometimes following their late spouse in death within a few months. As friends die off there are fewer and fewer with whom the elderly can communicate as peers. Coupled with the natural introversion present in the elderly, loneliness is all too common. The highest suicide rate is in elderly men living alone.

Accommodation

Elderly people are often forced to live in unsuitable accommodation owing to their poor socio-economic position. This may place them at considerable distance away from suitable shopping areas, access to transportation, and health services.

Independence

The result of the factors mentioned above is increasing dependency on others. This role reversal is very painful to the elderly and to those who are close to them.

Life

Contrary to expectations, the elderly are often not prepared for the end of life. This is encountered in the form of absence of wills and financial securities for the surviving spouse.

Styles of ageing

Some maintain that the elderly cope best if they accept the inevitability of ageing, a quieter life, and reduced social contact.

Others stress that the elderly, being aware of certain failing skills, must make all the more effort to counteract this deterioration in order to maintain a sense of purpose and satisfaction. The answer probably lies somewhere in between, and depends on factors such as personality type, cultural background, and former interests.

In practice, community workers will often find that ageing is dominated by anxiety and hypochondriasis, indecision, irritability and frustration, defiance, denial, and dependency.

Fortunately, some 70 per cent of individuals adapt constructively. Research has shown that, as a close friend and
'sounding-board', a community worker has a vital role to play
in alleviating these problems.

Conclusion

The best way to manage old age is not to wait for a cure but
rather to adopt a healthy life-style that prevents morbid
disease and preserves fitness, vigour, and independence. We
need to ensure that our surroundings are safe, that we have
enduring powers of attorney and living wills, and that we
limit inappropriate and inhumane terminal care. In all these
attempts however, we need the collective support in moral
and real terms not only of the community and of caregivers,
but also of those invested with power and responsibilities
that enable them to make changes that help the ageing population. Apart from the elderly themselves, their caregivers,
and the immediate community in contact with them, there is
very little awareness of the elderly and of their needs.

19 Cognitive disorders: delirium and dementia

Delirium

In the clinical setting, delirium is most frequently encountered in the 'confused patient'. The most common history is that of a sudden onset of inappropriate behaviour, disorientation, confusion, restlessness, or withdrawal in a patient who was completely 'intact' minutes or hours before. This condition was previously called 'acute organic brain syndrome'. It is a physical illness presenting with impaired consciousness, and needs immediate medical attention aimed at recognition of the cause of the syndrome, and if possible, reversal of it.

Making the diagnosis

Onset

This is acute, and there is a time-related connection with the cause. In the demented elderly, it more often occurs in the late afternoon and evening ('sundowning').

Symptoms

Attention
The patient cannot focus, and is therefore distractible and reacts indiscriminately to stimuli.

Orientation
Most patients are disorientated for time, place, and situation. They cannot give an account of recent events. They may know who and where they are if the surroundings are familiar.

Speech
Speech is often incoherent, inappropriate to the conversation, poor in content, fragmented, and the patient tends to skip between irrelevant issues. There may be paranoid ideation.

Memory
Memory for recent events is poor or 'patchy'.

Recognition and perception
Familiar voices, people, places, and objects may be misnamed. Misinterpretation of external stimuli (illusions) and false perceptions of the auditory, visual, and tactile senses (hallucinations) may be experienced.

Behaviour
Interaction with surroundings is disordered. Behaviour is inappropriate and sometimes aimless. Patients may be either restless, disinhibited, and agitated (hyperactive), or the reverse: slow, apathetic, and inattentive (hypoactive).

Affect
Emotions are inappropriate to the situation, and may encompass anger, fear, euphoria, or depression. The patient seems perplexed and out of touch and may alternate between uncontrollable laughter and crying, as if 'emotionally incontinent'.

Physiology

Autonomic symptoms such as sweating, tachycardia, tremor, anxiety, and tachypnoea may be present in cases of substance withdrawal delirium and the delirium of medical emergencies such as hypoglycaemia, hypoxia, systemic infections, and other toxic states.

Course

The onset is acute, and the disorder fluctuates over hours to days. It is usually reversible if the cause can be treated. Following recovery, the patient has a circumscribed amnesia, or only patchy recall for the period of delirium.

Note: People who take care of the elderly or in-patients can often observe the fluctuating course of the delirium better than a clinician seeing the patient for the first time. There may be a history of both lucid periods when the patient is in contact with his or her surroundings, and periods of confusion.

Common causes of delirium

Central nervous system disorders

Central nervous system disorders that could cause delirium are:
- epilepsy and post-ictal states;
- cerebrovascular causes such as stroke or subdural haematoma;
- concussion;
- infections such as encephalitis or meningitis; and
- tumours.

Drugs

Delirium can be caused by:
- prescribed drugs, such as anticholinergics, antihypertensives, anticonvulsants, antiparkinsonian and antipsychotic drugs, cardiac glycosides, H2-receptor antagonists (e.g. cimetidine, ranitidine), hypnotics, and steroids;
- alcohol;
- poison: carbon monoxide, heavy metals, and industrial poisons; and
- illegal drugs.

Systemic illnesses

Systemic causes of delirium include:
- urinary, HIV, and respiratory infections, malaria, and septicaemia;
- endocrine disorders (hypo- or hyper-): pituitary, adrenal, parathyroid, and thyroid; and
- metabolic disorders: hypo- or hyperglycaemia, uraemia, hepatic encephalopathy, and electrolyte disturbance.

Other causes:

Delirium can also be caused by:
- hypothermia;
- porphyria;
- deficiencies in vitamin B1, B12, nicotinic acid, or folate;
- post-operative states; and
- hypoxia or hypercarbia.

Medical management of delirium

Delirium is caused by a medical or substance-use disorder, and is a sign of deterioration in the patient's condition. The syndrome indicates impairment of consciousness and the patient needs urgent medical attention. The following aspects must be attended to:
- The patient must be safe. Delirious patients are often restless.
- Get the history from family or friends, and check for a Medic-Alert. Look for trauma, substance abuse, known medical conditions like diabetes and porphyria, and prescribed drugs.
- Check that the airway is clear, observe breathing rate, blood pressure, pulse, and temperature.
- Sniff the breath for intoxication and look for needle marks on arms, neck, and legs.
- Note pupil reactions and examine the patient for neuro-logical differences between the left and right sides of the body (reflexes, tone, pupil size, spontaneous movements), or unilateral neglect.
- Measure blood glucose with dextrostix.

If the physical examination confirms a toxic or neurological disorder, the patient should immediately be transferred to a medical emergency service. If possible, a slow intravenous drip with 5 per cent dextrose water should be set up. A severely intoxicated patient should lie on his or her side. A trained nurse should accompany the patient to ensure free breathing and should keep a suction apparatus at hand.

Contact the emergency service and give details. If the delirium appears to be the result of substance withdrawal, lorazepam 2–4 mg may be given intramuscularly (IM). If the patient is lucid enough to swallow safely, diazepam 5–15 mg may be administered orally for acute withdrawal symptoms. If the patient is agitated (overactive form of delirium), and a withdrawal state is not likely, haloperidol 5–10 mg may be administered IM for sedation. (Rather than over-sedate the patient, administer a small dose and repeat if necessary after twenty minutes.) In the elderly and the medically ill, doses should be lower.

If the examination confirms that the patient is stable:
- do a complete physical examination;
- do bedside blood and urine tests; and
- start appropriate special investigations.

Special investigations

First line
- Blood: full blood count, ESR, glucose, urea and electrolytes, liver functions and thyroid functions.
- Urine: Multistix, MSU sample for culture, toxicology screening for cannabis, methaqualone, opiates, and benzodiazepines.
- ECG.
- Chest X-ray.
- CSF examination: chemistry, microbiology, culture, IgG index, and syphilis serology.
- EEG and brain scan only if the cause of the delirium is still unknown and CNS pathology needs to be ruled out.

The patient should be admitted and supportive measures instituted. Regular observations, intake and output monitoring, and appropriate treatment of the cause should be initiated. In very young or aged and other delirium-prone patients, clinicians must remember that mild infections, dehydration, and non-threatening disorders may cause delirium, and unnecessary investigations that cause patient discomfort and delay the start of treatment should be avoided.

Second line

- Blood: serum folate and B12, HIV antibodies, cardiac enzymes, blood gases, auto-antibody screen, blood cultures, calcium, and phosphate.
- Cranial computerized tomography.

Management of withdrawal states

Most of the substance withdrawal states respond well to long-acting benzodiazepines like diazepam. Alcohol withdrawal is the most severe and dangerous of the withdrawal syndromes. With short-acting drugs like alcohol, withdrawal symptoms are worst during the first forty-eight hours and the patient may need large doses of a drug like diazepam in the early stages of withdrawal. Diazepam 5–10 mg may be given orally three to six-hourly during this phase. Lorazepam 2–4 mg IM may supplement the oral diazepam.

Note: Delirium may have more than one cause. A patient in alcohol withdrawal must be examined thoroughly to exclude other life-threatening disorders such as infection, trauma, blood loss, vitamin deficiencies, and metabolic disorders.

Alcoholics must always be administrered vitamin B1 (thiamine) 100 mg IM daily for the first five to seven days to prevent Wernicke's encephalopathy (delirium, ataxia, nystagmus, and cranial nerve III, IV, and VI ophthalmoplegia). If an alcoholic in withdrawal is being given a glucose-containing drip, the thiamine should be given intravenously.

Dementia

Dementia is an impairment in memory with associated cognitive deficits that in turn affect personality and intellect, as well as social and occupational functioning in an alert patient. Memory impairment is the inability to learn new information and to recall previously learned information. Other cognitive deficits include:

- aphasia (language disturbance);
- apraxia (inability to carry out motor activities despite intact motor function);
- agnosia (failure to recognize or identify objects despite intact sensory function); and
- disturbance in executive functioning (i.e. planning, organizing, sequencing, and abstracting).

Prevalence

The prevalence of dementia in the general population is 5 per cent. It rises with age, from approximately 3 per cent among sixty-year-olds to 5 per cent at sixty-five and 20 per cent at eighty. A maximum prevalence of 30 per cent occurs on reaching the ninety-year-old range.

Aetiology

The syndrome of dementia becomes a diagnosis once the cause of the dementia has been established, often only definitively at post-mortem examination. Alzheimer's disease accounts for some 50 per cent of all cases of dementia, vascular dementia for 20 per cent, and mixed causes (i.e. both Alzheimer's and vascular) for 15 per cent. The remainder consists of dementia induced by alcoholism (5 per cent), while dementia associated with other causes (such as HIV dementia, brain injury, Parkinson's disease, neurosyphilis, hypothyroidism, tumours, pellagra, folate and vitamin B12 deficiencies) accounts for the remaining 10 per cent. Note that HIV dementia is steadily on the increase. Dementia is almost invariably progressive but its profound psychosocial effects may respond to intervention, as may the causes hastening the disease process. Early diagnosis is therefore very important.

Diagnostic assessment

Firstly, it must be established whether dementia is in fact present. This may be difficult since the individual's reaction to the illness, the presence of drugs, physical illness, emotional upheavals, and depression may all complicate the picture. Collateral information from a spouse, family, or friends is essential. Patients must also be asked to bring their spectacles and/or hearing-aids, past medical records, and current medication to the interview. Questions addressed to informants should centre around the following points.

Memory impairment

This must be in excess of the so-called 'dodderiness', 'benign senescent forgetfulness' or 'age-associated memory impairment' that is found in some 30 per cent of all elderly people. In other words, the forgetfulness must be seen to interfere with usual daily functioning. Articles are mislaid, faces not recognized, disorientation for time or place occurs, and statements need to be repeated. Initially the patient with dementia has difficulty in learning new information (short-term memory), but later on long-term memory is also affected. Increasingly the person lives in the past.

Personality changes

This usually involves an accentuation of former personality traits, such as histrionic, impulsive, aggressive, or paranoid tendencies. Less commonly, an alteration of the personality occurs, in that the 'shadow' or the 'hidden side' of the person comes to the fore. Eventually a normally active individual becomes increasingly apathetic and withdrawn, with a narrowing of social involvement. The personality loses its sparkle and the individual is no longer herself or himself. The patient may become self-centred, hypochondriacal, argumentative, self-neglectful, and can be said to have entered into a 'second childhood'. Impaired judgement and impulse control may be observed, for example social disinhibition, clumsy shoplifting or other theft, inappropriate money spending, and exhibitionism.

Intellectual impairment

People with dementia may stop reading, listening to the radio, watching television, or occupying themselves constructively. They are no longer able to grasp the meaning of a conversation, and have to be addressed in 'simple' language. Language may become vague, stereotyped, and imprecise. Dysphasia (ranging from an inability to find the right word to mumbling speech or jargon dysphasia) may manifest.

Emotional changes

Sensitivity, interest, and affection may disappear, and the subtle interchange of feelings and understanding that play so important a part in any relationship become distressingly absent. The patient may be described as being 'cold'. The mood is not usually depressed – emotional superficiality is more common. Occasional bouts of irritability occur.

Investigations

Once the presence of dementia has been established, the aetiology and possible presence of reversible factors need to be considered. This is obtained on history, physical examination concentrating on neurological deficit, observations, and, where indicated, investigations.

Generally, in typical or advanced cases of dementia, investigations have little to offer towards diagnosis and treatment. Furthermore, investigations cannot be performed routinely, and are more likely to yield a positive result when:

- the patient is under sixty-five years of age;
- the dementia has been of recent and rapid onset;
- the course of the disease fluctuates markedly; and
- the physical examination reveals a neurological deficit.

Functional assessment

This is mandatory in order to plan future care. The aim is to assess the degree of disability as well as the retained abilities so that the patient can be helped to maintain the best possible quality of life within the community.

It involves the assessment of:

- mobility;
- ability to communicate needs;
- ability to relate to others;
- ability to wash and dress self;
- ability to feed self;
- control of bladder and bowels; and
- presence of aggression and other socially unacceptable behaviour.

Social assessment

This determines the patient's present social functioning and ability to care for himself or herself. Assess the:

- need for supervision;
- ability to prepare meals;
- ability to go shopping;
- ability to do housework; and
- compliance with medication.

The social assessment takes into consideration accommodation, employment, and economic resources, and evaluates the degree of available social support. Once the above information has been gathered, each patient's future can be projected and planned with regard to care and placement.

Medical management of dementia

The above assessments will indicate the correct management for a specific patient. At present there is no cure for Alzheimer's disease and most other dementias. The treatment of dementia is aimed at reversible factors and symptom alleviation such as:

- Anxiety, restlessness and psychotic symptoms, which may be medicated as outlined in Table 19.1
- When a delirium (usually due to urinary tract infection or bronchopneumonia) is superimposed on an already existing dementia, the drug treatment should commence at a higher dosage level as specified in Table 19.1.
- Currently only the drugs donepezil (Aricept) and rivastigimine (Exelon) have been shown to improve or

slow down the dementing process, but this is often a temporary effect.

- In the early stages of dementia 10 to 20 per cent of patients will suffer from depression. However, among patients with vascular and Parkinson's disease dementias the incidence may approach 30 per cent. While depression usually responds well to antidepressant medication, this is usually not the case in patients with a mini-mental state examination (MMSE) score of less than 22, where the so-called 'depression' is in fact dementia.
- Reduction of the formation of platelet thrombi by administering salicyclic acid (half a Disprin, i.e. 150 mg daily) is the prescribed treatment for transient ischaemic attacks occurring in vascular dementias.
- Control of hypertension, taking into account raised age-acceptable blood pressures.
- Control of diabetes, noting that in asymptomatic diabetics blood glucose levels of up to 15 mmol/l are acceptable.
- Reduction of smoking, aiming at fewer than five cigarettes per day with meals and teas.
- Reduction of alcohol consumption to the equivalent of three tots of spirits a day.

Should the patient not be controlled on the above regimens, referral to a more specialized unit is indicated. Judicious use of the correct psychotropic medications can make all the difference in making the patient acceptable in the community for care by the family at home, as opposed to permanent placement in an old-age home.

Table 19.1 Treatment schedule for sedation

Haloperidol

- 0.5 mg twice daily
- Increase the dose to 0,75 mg, 1.0 mg and 1.5 mg twice daily if necessary, for daytime control. Wait a day or two between increases.

Together with

Table 19.1 continued

Oral *Zuclopenthixol*

- 2 mg twice daily and 4 mg at night

Occasionally, oral chlorpromazine 20–50 mg, or intramuscular lorazepam, 2–4 mg or haloperidol, 2,5 mg may initially be required for control.

Table 19.2 Differentiating features of delirium, depression, and dementia

	Delirium	**Depression**	**Dementia**
Onset	Rapid (hours to days).	Rapid (weeks to months).	Gradual (years).
Course	Wide fluctuations, may continue for weeks if cause not found.	May be self-limited or may become chronic without treatment.	Chronic, slow but continuous decline.
Level of consciousness	Fluctuates from hyper-alert to difficult to arouse.	Normal.	Normal.
Orientation	Patient is disoriented, confused.	Patient may seem disoriented.	Patient is disoriented, confused.
Affect	Fluctuating.	Sad, depressed, worried, guilty.	Labile, apathy in later stages.
Attention	Always impaired.	Difficulty concentrating, patient may check and recheck all actions.	May be intact, patient may focus on one thing for long periods.

Table 19.2 continued

Sleep	Always disturbed.	Disturbed, excess sleeping or insomnia, especially early-morning waking.	Usually normal.
Behaviour	Agitated, restless.	Patient may be fatigued, apathetic, may occasionally be agitated.	Patient may be agitated or apathetic, may wander.
Speech	Sparse or rapid, patient incoherent.	Flat, sparse, may have understand-able outbursts.	Sparse or rapid, repetitive; patient may be incoherent.
Memory	Impaired, especially for recent events.	Varies day-to-day, slow recall, often short-term deficit.	Impaired, especially for recent events.
Cognition	Disordered reasoning.	May seem impaired.	Disordered reasoning and calculation.
Thought content	Incoherent, confused, delusions, stereotyped.	Negative, hypochondriac, thoughts of death, paranoid.	Disorganized, rich content, delusional, paranoid.
Perception	Misinterpreta-tions; illusions; hallucinations.	Distorted, patient may have auditory hallucinations, negative inter-pretation of people and events.	No change.

Table 19.2 continued

Judgment	Poor.	Poor.	Poor, socially inappropriate behaviour.
Insight	May be present in lucid moments.	May be impaired.	Absent.
Performance on mental state exams	Poor but variable, improves during lucid moments and with recovery.	Memory impaired, calculation, drawing following directions, usually not impaired, frequent 'I don't know' answers.	Consistently poor, progressively worsens; patient attempts to answer all questions.

Nursing management: delirium and dementia

Patients that suffer from delirium or dementia have altered thought processes. *Note: the primary nursing goal for these patients is reorientation (as far as possible) to reality.*

Older people, especially those suffering from dementia can be very sensitive to the side-effects of medication, and nurses should watch for these. Some patients who suffer from dementia are not able to live in open communities and may need institutionalization. This is a problem as there are very few suitable facilities. In less severe cases it may be possible to establish day-care centres where patients with dementia can be cared for during the day.

Table 19.3 summarizes some useful nursing interventions that may help to orientate the patient with regards to time, place, and person.

Nurses should educate families about these guidelines so that they can also help to support and orientate the client.

Table 19.3 Recommended nursing interventions for delirium and dementia

- Orientate the patient with regards to time by making a clock, a calendar, a daily newspaper, and current magazines available.
- Provide access to radio or television and evaluate the patient's interpretation of the broadcasted material.
- Refer to specific dates, times, and events. This referral to specific times can coincide with your programme in the clinic. For example: 'Mr. Peters your next appointment will be on the 20th June at noon.'
- Provide access to, and encourage the patient's participation in, current community or hospital activities and functions.
- Maintain a consistent time schedule with the patient.
- Give the patient a copy of his or her monthly schedule and go through it together.
- Tell the patient where he or she is: identify the clinic, the date, the time, and repeat all information as needed.
- Have the patient explore and investigate his or her room. Designate the patient's room with a nameplate on the door. Educate the family on this to guide and support the patient.
- Explain sounds the patient might hear, for example the closing of the elevator door, carts being wheeled through the hall, and the paging and ward intercom systems.
- Identify personnel by title – nurse, physician, and nursing assistant.
- Let the family provide night-lights.
- Maintain familiar surroundings (patients should have their own clothes, possessions, and routines).
- Address the patient by name and title. Instruct staff members to address the patient by name and to state their relationship to him or her.
- Label clothing and possessions with the name the patient uses at home.
- Explore the patient's perceptions of him- or herself and reinforce reality when appropriate.
- Plan and implement a consistent approach.

Drug therapy in the elderly

Note that elderly patients with visual and intellectual impairment make frequent errors in taking their medication. The elderly may also take non-prescription drugs such as laxatives, painkillers, and sleeping tablets. Age-related changes in drug absorption, body composition, metabolism, and kidney function render elderly people more sensitive to the adverse effects of drugs. Dosage should be adjusted on the basis of response. The minimum number of drugs should be prescribed, taken in as few doses per day as possible, and instructions should be clear.

Follow-up, with response, adverse effect, and compliance checks is important. Drug interactions and adverse effects are often causes of delirium in the elderly. The patient should be admitted, drugs should be rationalized and drug education should be provided. Compliance should be regularly monitored by the people who take care of the infirm elderly.

Mini-mental state examination (MMSE)

This is a very useful instrument, which can be used, particularly for distinguishing dementia from pseudo-dementia. A score of below 24 for literate patients and below 20 for illiterate patients is indicative of dementia. Usually, there is no time limit in completing this.

Table 19.4 Mini-mental state examination (MMSE)

Orientation	Score	Points
1 What is the year?	_____	1
season?	_____	1
month?	_____	1
day?	_____	1
date?	_____	1
2 Where are we?		
country?	_____	1
province?	_____	1

Table 19.4 continued

	Score	Points
town or city?	_____	1
hospital?	_____	1
ward?	_____	1

Registration

3 Name three objects, taking one second to say each. Then ask the patient to repeat all three once you have said them. Give one point for each correct answer. Rehearse the answers until the patient learns all three.   _____ 3

Attention and calculation

4 Serial sevens. Give one point for each correct answer. Stop after five answers. Alternate: Spell 'world' backwards, or 'herfs' (for Afrikaans-speaking patients).   _____ 5

Recall

5 Ask for the names of the three objects learned in question 3 above. Give one point for each correct answer.   _____ 3

Language

6 Point to a pencil and a watch. Have the patient name them as you point.   _____ 2

7 Have the patient follow a three-stage command: 'Take this paper in your right hand. Fold the paper in half. Put the paper on the floor.'   _____ 1

8 Have the patient repeat 'No ifs, ands, or buts' or 'Nog vis, nog vlees, nog voël' (Afrikaans-speaking patients).   _____ 1

9 Have the patient read and obey the following: 'Close your eyes.' (Write it in large letters.)   _____ 1

10 Have the patient write a sentence of his or her choice. (The sentence should contain a subject

Table 19.4 continued

	Score	Points
and an object, and should make sense. Ignore spelling errors when scoring.)	_____	1
11 Have the patient copy the design printed below. (Give one point if all sides and the angles are preserved and if the intersecting sides form a diamond shape.)	_____	1

Date: ....   **Total:** _____ 30

20 Psychotic disorders: schizophrenia

Patients with psychotic disorders such as schizophrenia are out of touch with reality. Their behaviour is often very bizarre and their thoughts disturbed. They may suffer from delusions (false beliefs) and they may hallucinate (usually hearing or seeing things that aren't there).

Psychotic patients typically:

- hear voices;
- see objects that no one else can see;
- have strange physical complaints (such as snakes in the stomach);
- have difficulties with thought-processes (such as thinking and concentrating); and
- are confused, bewildered, and lack concentration.

The families often ask for help because this behaviour is strange and often frightening.

Note: Patients who are disorientated for time, place, and person and who have memory impairment are probably suffering from delirium and need urgent medical attention.

Schizophrenia

Schizophrenia, which literally means splitting of the mind, is the most common psychotic disorder. Schizophrenic disorders are characterized by:

- distorted thinking and perception;
- flat or inappropriate affect, i.e. blunted emotions;
- auditory hallucinations;
- ambivalence and disturbance of volition (lack of purpose); and
- catatonia and other abnormal or disorganized behaviour.

The onset of the disorder may be acute or insidious.

Aetiology

The cause of schizophrenia is as yet unknown. Schizophrenia comprises a group of disorders with heterogeneous causes. Some theories are:

- *Stress-diathesis model*: According to this model a person may have the vulnerability (diathesis) which, when they undergo some stressful environmental influence, allows the symptoms of schizophrenia to develop.
- *Dopamine hypothesis*: This theory suggests that the symptoms of schizophrenia are the result of too much central dopaminergic activity in the brain.
- *Genetic contribution*: Family studies strongly suggest that there is a genetic component to schizophrenia. The prevalence in the general population is approximately 1 per cent. Children with one schizophrenic parent have a 12 per cent chance of developing schizophrenia, while children who have two schizophrenic parents have a 40 per cent chance.

Symptoms reported by family and friends

The patient's family and friends usually note a drastic change in the patient's behaviour. The patient behaves bizarrely. There is withdrawal and a lack of interest and drive, with deterioration in personal hygiene. The patient's behaviour is unexpected and family and friends are puzzled.

Physical examination

Usually no abnormalities are found. However, factors such as substance abuse (for instance cannabis), or medical conditions such as epilepsy or pellagra, either of which may be the cause of a psychotic condition, should be excluded.

Mental state: features

General description

The patient's general appearance can be affected in many ways and may be dishevelled and agitated, or withdrawn and mute.

Disturbance of emotions

Affect is said to be flat or blunted where the patient expresses little or no emotion, or inappropriate emotion. Note that blunted affect may be a symptom of the illness itself, the Parkinsonian side-effects of antipsychotic medication, or depression.

Perceptual disturbance

Auditory hallucinations are most common but there may also be visual, olfactory, gustatory, and tactile hallucinations. The voices are often threatening, accusatory, or insulting. Two or more voices may converse among themselves, or may comment on the patient's life or behaviour, or direct orders at the patient (command hallucinations).

Disturbance of thought form

Thinking is frequently incomprehensible to others and appears illogical. Disorders of thought form include:
- *loosening of associations* (derailment) where the ideas are unrelated and shift from one topic to another in a completely unrelated way; and
- *flight of ideas* where there is rapid shifting from one idea to another.

Speech is incoherent and incomprehensible:

- The patient may give irrelevant answers where the answer has no bearing on the question.
- There may be neologisms (where patients coin new words that may have a symbolic meaning for them), over-inclusiveness, blocking, and echolalia.
- There may be *poverty of speech* (where the patient speaks very little).
- There may be *poverty of content* (where the patient speaks a normal amount but conveys little information).

Disturbance of thought content

The most important disorder of thought content is delusion. The delusions occur frequently and may be bizarre (a false idea that is totally implausible in the person's culture, such as thought broadcasting). In *persecutory* delusions patients believe, for example, that others are spying on them, spreading false rumours, or planning to harm or kill them (for example, by poisoning their food).

Delusions of *reference* occur where patients attach special and unusual meaning, usually negative, to events, objects, or other people. Examples are perceptions that they are being referred to by other people, or on television, or that when something is broadcast (for example, certain music) it has a special meaning, such as that one should stop work or start dancing. Delusions of reference are also referred to as *explanatory* delusions or delusions of *interpretation*.

Certain delusions are more common in schizophrenia than in other psychotic disorders. These include:

- *Thought broadcasting:* The delusion that thoughts are broadcast from the patient's head to the outside world, so that others can also hear them.
- *Thought insertion:* The delusion that the thoughts are not the patient's own but have been implanted in his or her mind.
- *Thought withdrawal:* The delusion that thoughts have been removed from the patient's mind.
- *Delusions of control:* The delusion that thoughts, feelings, impulses, or acts are not the patient's own, but are imposed or controlled by an external power or authority, for example by X-rays.

Other delusions that may present are *somatic, grandiose, religious,* and *nihilistic* delusions.

Orientation and memory

As with other psychotic patients, schizophrenic patients are usually oriented to time, place, and person. If this is not the case, the possibility of a neurological disorder or substance abuse should be investigated.

Medical management

The acutely psychotic patient must be referred either to hospital or to the community psychiatric services for further treatment. When the patient has been discharged, he or she needs to remain on treatment with antipsychotics. These can be given in tablet form, to be taken daily by the patient. If there is a problem with compliance, then long-acting injectable antipsychotic medication can be given, monthly or two-weekly, depending on the patient's condition. They should be stabilized before being referred to the primary health care nurse and the nurse should be given some idea of how long the patient needs to be on medication. They should be seen by the nurse at least every three months if stable, more often, if not. They should be referred back to community psychiatric services for an annual review or if they relapse.

Drug treatment

Several drugs are available that can be used to sedate the acutely psychotic or aggressive patient. Remember to do as much physical examination as possible before sedating. If the patient is physically ill, i.e. acute cardiac problems, then give lower doses of medication.

The following drugs are available in South Africa:
- Haloperidol (Serenace) 5 mg orally, IMI or IVI (slowly) or: 0,5–2 mg if the patient is medically ill. This is the treatment of choice if the patient is medically ill.
- Zuclopenthixol (Clopixol Acuphase) 50–150 mg IMI stat. The effect will last two to three days (Must be kept in fridge).

- Clothiapine (Etomine) 40–80 mg orally, IMI or IVI (slowly). Can be repeated up to 160 mg in 24 hours. At present, this is not on the EDL (see Chapter 25) for PHC, but may be available in some clinics.
- Diazepam (Valium) 10 mg orally, IVI (slowly) or rectally (slowly). Use these in patients with epilepsy, or alcohol withdrawal, or other drug withdrawal states.
- Lorazepam (Ativan) IMI or IVI 0,5–2 mg (must be kept in fridge). Also useful for the medically ill.
- Chlorpromazine (Largactil) 50–100 mg orally. Should not be given by injection. It is painful, causes local inflammation, but more importantly, can suddenly drop BP to dangerously low levels.

Some of these drugs may not be available in your area, but at least diazepam and one other should be available.

Note: Do not give combinations of antipsychotics. This increases the likelihood of dangerous side-effects. However, the combination of an antipsychotic and a benzodiazepine can be useful in the acutely psychotic patient, e.g. haloperidol together with lorazepam or diazepam.

Rehabilitation or community support

Patients need to know where to go to when they have problems. They may need assistance with finding employment or being trained for work, or sheltered employment. Training in various skills may be useful. They are entitled to a disability grant from the State.

Table 20.1 Antipsychotics and benzodiazepines

Antipsychotics	Benzodiazepines
Chlorpromazine (Largactil)	Diazepam (Valium)
Haloperidol (Serenace)	Lorazepam (Ativan)
Zuclopenthixol (Clopixol Acuphase)	Clonazepam (Rivotril)
Fluphenazine (Modecate)	Oxazepam (Serepax)
Trifluoperazine (Stelazine)	
Clothiapine (Etomine)	

Referral back to hospital when indicated

When patients become acutely psychotic and cannot be managed at home by increasing medication, they should be referred back to hospital or to the local community psychiatric clinic until they are stable again. Occasionally, patients are chronically unmanageable, and if there are facilities, they may need to be institutionalized.

Counselling the family

Patients with psychotic illness often lack insight into their illness and may refuse to take treatment. The nurse should explain the treatment programme to them several times, and in the most supportive way possible. Families can often assist here, but they must also be educated about the condition. They need to know:

- that this often strange or frightening behaviour can be treated and is symptomatic of mental illness;
- that their support and understanding is crucial for compliance with treatment and effective follow-up care; and
- that the acute symptoms (hallucinations, agitation, severe delusions, and aggression) often resolve with treatment, but can recur; compliance with the treatment regimen is therefore very important.

Families must understand the need for medication, the course of the illness, and the outcome. Family members often feel very guilty when someone in their family becomes ill in this way. They may feel ashamed. They need to be reassured and supported. Community education is important so that these patients can be understood, if not accepted by the community. The nurse will need to do the following:

- Offer information about the illness. This will contribute to the reduction of the stigma of mental illness. Do not force information on people. Also try to remain as neutral as possible. A good way to do this is to say 'I have information for you about this illness, do you want me to tell you about it?' or 'I could give you a lot more information, are you interested?'

- Educate families on how to handle patients if they relapse (see Table 20.2) or need emergency treatment. Tell family members what to expect of the patient in terms of their functioning. Very often, family members think that the mentally ill person is lazy and may expect too much from him or her. Some mental illnesses affect people's functioning.

Prepare families for handling a mentally ill person at home. The most important aspects of this preparation are the following:

- *Discuss feelings*: Find out how each person in the family feels about looking after the sick relative. Listen carefully to everyone and be sure to reflect feelings and communicate understanding.
- *Discuss changes*: Ask the family members how they think having a mentally ill person in the home will affect their lives. What changes will they need to make? Be careful not to judge negative feelings in the family. If you handle this session correctly the family may feel relieved and able to handle the situation with your support. Let them know that you understand their situation and are there to listen if they need to talk.
- *Discuss expectations*: The family should know what the patient can and cannot do. Part of the preparation involves discussing rehabilitation and how to enable the patient to reach his or her functional potential.
- *Discuss support systems*: Tell the family about the importance of having breaks from the patient, acknowledging their own needs, and trying to deal with guilt feelings. Focus on the long-term impact that looking after sick relatives can have on careers. Encourage families to consider ways of having breaks from the responsibility, sharing their feelings with each other, and finding support networks for themselves.

Table 20.2 Management of acute agitation in psychotic patients

The family should support the treatment plan and understand what to do during acute episodes of agitation or excitement:

- Assess and secure the safety of the patient and those caring for him or her.
- Ensure that the patient's basic needs (food and drink) are met.
- Do not argue with abnormal beliefs.
- Ensure that dangerous behaviour or severe agitation receives close supervision or hospitalization. (Families may need help managing disruptive and threatening behaviour.)
- Institute legal measures if patients refuse treatment.
- Encourage resumption of normal activities after symptoms improve. (Unreasonable expectations are harmful, but the patient should be allowed to function at the highest level of his or her ability in work or daily activities.)
- Avoid confrontation or criticism unless it is necessary to prevent harmful or disruptive behaviour.

Summary

The following table summarizes the management of the chronic patient in the PHC setting.

Table 20.3 Summary of PHC management for schizophrenic patients

1 During the patient's visit always check how stable his or her present environment is
Does he or she receive the disability grant?
Is the patient on good terms with his or her family?
Does he or she experience any side-effects?
Does he or she have any problems to discuss?
Does he or she abuse substances?

2 Check for symptoms of psychosis

Does the patient:

Hear voices?

Believe that people are ganging up against him or her?

Feel elated or depressed?

Describe any unusual subjective experiences?

3 Continue with prescribed treatment

If the patient has just been discharged from hospital check if he or she receives major doses of oral treatment together with IMI treatment. If so, then very slowly decrease the oral medication and if possible refer to the doctor for review.

4 If a patient or relatives complain about uncomfortable side-effects

Provide education on management of uncomfortable side-effects (see Chapter 25) and either treat with respective drugs Akineton and Disipal, or decrease the medication slowly over a period of time while referring the patient to a doctor for review.

5 Never discontinue

Only if IMI medication like Modecate or Clopixol has side-effects that are intolerably severe should it be discontinued. Always encourage patients and relatives to stick with the injectable antipsychotics.

6 Referral points

Make sure that the telephone number of the closest secondary referral point or nearest psychiatrist are readily available, so that they can be consulted if necessary.

21 Substance abuse

Substance abuse poses a serious health and financial threat to both the individual and the community. No person intentionally becomes substance dependent, and addiction must be approached with empathy and energy.

Substance abuse has many causes, and nurses need to understand the interaction between the vulnerable person (often an adolescent), socio-economic stressors, societal changes, and cultural norms. The realities of drug availability, peer pressure, pressure to achieve, and the collapse of family systems must be appreciated. The use of alcohol in our community has been accepted for centuries and a substantial percentage of the community can use alcohol quite regularly without serious social or personal consequences.

Every potential patient moves through the phases of drug or alcohol experimentation, use, abuse, and dependence. Although the end results of alcohol and drug abuse are often identical, there are differences that warrant separate therapeutic approaches to the two types of abuse. Experimentation with and use of alcohol are socially accepted, while drug use is usually illegal and is seen as deviant behaviour.

As with alcohol, young people and children may experiment with drugs. Most of them drop out of the 'drug scene' almost immediately. A smaller percentage may become social users of drugs. Use may become abuse, and because drug use is criminal, a secretive, isolated life-style may develop. This subculture may lead to self-defeating behaviour, with sexual promiscuity and stealing in order to secure the money to satisfy a growing need for expensive drugs. The last phase of drug dependence is total addiction, when addicts will spend all their time and talents on securing a supply for intoxication. They miss out on normal developmental tasks and become ill-equipped for the challenges of adult life. Opportunistic infections, trauma, arrests, and overdose may have end-of-the-road consequences.

Substance abuse is a medical disorder and can be successfully treated, which helps not only the individual but often also the family and the community.

Definitions

Experimentation

While trying out once or on a few occasions, usually in the peer group context, an individual may suffer the consequences of intoxication. Experimentation is common and, if recognized, should be confronted immediately and openly.

Use

With social use, not constantly but regularly, the individual may suffer the consequences of intoxication. Regular use of illegal drugs may lead to arrests.

Abuse

With regular intoxication, substance use occurs out of the social context, the person is intoxicated during the daytime, and may suffer the consequences of intoxication in the form of drunken driving arrests, marital discord, problems in the workplace, and deterioration of health. This phase is characterized by excuses, promises, and denial.

Dependence

Following abuse, tolerance develops and when the substance is discontinued, withdrawal symptoms occur (physical dependence). Psychological dependence refers to the repeated psychological need for the effect (the 'kick' or 'escape') offered by intoxication.

The therapist

(*Note:* In under-resourced circumstances the nurse may have to fulfil the role of the therapist.) Few successful primary prevention programmes have been implemented in our society. Poverty, educational deprivation, family pathology, and a lack of social support systems render them ineffective. There is also a high 'escape' percentage, even after completion of a good programme. Early detection of substance abuse and appropriate confrontation of the patient are therefore of the utmost importance. Therapists must accept the substance abuser as a patient in need, and must be confident and persistent enough to confront the problem. The motivation for confrontation is 'I care for my patient and I am not afraid to confront him or her with the reality that substance abuse may be the cause of his or her physical, psychological, or social problems'.

Therapists must be able to recognize the early signs of substance abuse and must confirm the abuse through collateral information from the patient's family, friends, or colleagues. Confrontation must be followed by a plan of action aimed at healing. Therapists must not be discouraged by the patient's refusal of help, and should encourage the family and employer to stop enabling the patient and to take a caring but tough stand. Therapists should accept and internalize the following, so as to become comfortable with themselves, the patient, and the road of healing ahead:

- Patients may be very demanding when intoxicated or in withdrawal.

- Patients who are substance abusers always *minimize* ('I hardly drink'), *rationalize* ('It makes me creative and relaxes me'), *project* ('I drink because of my wife or boss), *intellectualize* ('I know all about alcohol'), and *deny* ('I do not use drugs at all').
- Patients are not self-motivated and co-operation may be poor.
- Patients may relapse.
- Patients tend to view themselves as *victims* of external problems.
- Patients will try to *manipulate* the therapist for protection.

Therapeutic frustration may lead to retribution, rejection, or ignoring the patient's needs, while therapeutic perseverance may result in a therapeutic alliance, shared responsibility, and a plan of action and hope. It is important not to become isolated as a therapist: consult colleagues and team members.

The patient

No one becomes an addict on purpose. Every patient has sufficient personal, social, occupational, financial, and other problems that can be put forward as reasons for the development and likely continuation of substance abuse. At the start of therapy, patients are seldom able to come to grips with their personal vulnerability and limitations and many will therefore externalize the problem. Typically, every patient moves through the following stages:

- I have no problem.
- I have a problem, but I can control it without help.
- Maybe I am dependent. I am running out of excuses. I am in trouble. I must stop.
- See, I have stopped.
- Stop, start, stop, start.
- Sober, I am limited. I must now take responsibility. I need help. I must change my life-style. What are the pitfalls of intoxication, what should I avoid? I have changed my atti-

tude toward my future. Intoxication is not okay. I am not lonely anymore, there are others like me.
- I made it! It was not that difficult. I think I can use the substance socially without abuse. I have learnt my lesson.
- Relapse.

It should be clear that, during the first five stages, the motivation does not come from the patient, but from his or her environment (family, friends, place of work, and therapist). Repeated empathic but firm confrontation, followed by a plan of action, may initiate the healing process.

The family

Young people who consume alcohol are part of mainstream society, and abuse may be accepted for years. 'Enabling' by a spouse, children, doctor, and friends poses a severe problem. Early confrontation with resultant early intervention does not take place. To 'enable' a person's addiction means to make excuses, cover up, accept, endure, be bullied or manipulated into silence, take over his or her duties, or become the helpless victim of the alcohol abuser, thereby making it possible for these individuals to continue their drinking behaviour.

Recovery

Make it impossible for the substance abuser to continue his or her self-defeating behaviour. Be kind but firm. Do not be afraid of your patient; yielding to unrealistic demands, threats, and promises will enable your patient and the situation will continue unchanged. Identify the symptoms of early abuse and confront them at an early stage. Connect the presenting problems to the substance abuse. Point out the disadvantages of abuse and the advantages of sobriety. Formulate a plan of action. A therapist who is unable to motivate the patient should allow him or her to re-accept responsibility, but maintain hope and repeat the exercise at the next consultation.

Dealing with addicts

Nurses need to be able to recognize the signs of alcoholism (see p. 232) and drug abuse (see individual substances from p. 235), identify the stages the patients go through, and plan intervention programmes.

It is also important that nurses clarify their own feelings about alcoholism and drug addiction and are able to make an objective assessment of the patient. They should reflect on how their feelings and beliefs affect their interaction with the patient. Nurses might feel like failures if their patients don't recover soon. This needs to be addressed.

After recognition comes reaction:

- Report the signs and symptoms to the medical doctor and, together with the patient, work out a plan to address his or her needs.
- Don't allow the patient to manipulate you. Set firm limits and don't ignore the patient's demands. Listen to the patient and don't surrender control.
- Don't pass judgements and don't impose your values on the patient.
- The most direct way of dealing with a patient is to ask the patient about his or her drinking or drug habits, for instance 'How much alcohol do you drink a day?'
- Use your confrontational skills in dealing with the patient. This will help the patient to acknowledge the problem and avoid denial.

The following signs may indicate a relapse:

- exhaustion;
- fatigue;
- negative talking;
- dishonesty – unnecessary deceit;
- impatience;
- argumentativeness;
- depression;
- frustration;
- self-pity;
- irritability;

- overconfidence;
- complacency;
- expecting too much from others;
- blaming, shifting responsibility;
- use of mood-altering chemicals;
- unobtainable goals;
- concentrating on life problems;
- promises ('It's over, it won't happen again');
- feeling omnipotent; and
- having all the answers.

Treatment options

If the patient can be motivated, establish whether he or she will be prepared to undergo withdrawal symptoms (tremors, palpitations, sweating, anxiety, cravings). Admit the patient to a local hospital and detoxify (see individual substances). After withdrawal, motivate for further treatment. The following treatment options may be available:
- in-patient rehabilitation programmes;
- out-patient rehabilitation programmes;
- community-based self-help groups;
- community-based self-help groups for the families of addicts; and
- network therapy, i.e. the therapist, patient, spouse, child, family, friend, or supervisor form a network; this network takes part in a rehabilitation programme on an out-patient basis and provides therapeutic intervention, observation, and monitoring in daily life.

Note: Every primary health care therapist should have a list of the available resources in the relevant community, for instance:
- twelve-step programmes such as Alcoholics Anonymous or Narcotics Anonymous;
- other specialized programmes focusing on in-patient treatment like Houghton House, Dot's Plot, Crescent Clinic, Stepping Stones, Hillcrest Manor;
- medically-based in-patient treatment;

- out-patient treatment;
- the South African National Council for Alcohol and Drug Rehabilitation (SANCA);
- detoxification wards in hospitals; and
- specialized detoxification units in hospitals.

Watch for complications

During withdrawal, a patient who is seriously debilitated may have any of these potentially lethal complications:
- coronary problems;
- upper respiratory problems;
- liver failure;
- severe electrolyte imbalance; and
- convulsions

Observe the patient closely and inform the doctor immediately of any change in his or her condition.

Alcohol

Early recognition

- Regular physical complaints, for instance gastro-intestinal problems, hypertension, and trauma.
- Regular complaints of anxiety and depression with a positive alcohol history.
- Regular absence from work, and requests for medical certificates for vague physical complaints.
- Conflict in the family and place of work.
- Contact with the police.
- Physical examination: redness of the face and palms, enlarged liver, hypertension, gynaecomastia and withdrawal symptoms such as sweating, tremor, and tachycardia.
- History of alcohol abuse obtained from the family or supervisor.

Early and, if necessary, repeated confrontation

- Be empathic but firm.
- Confront the patient with facts and reality.
- Offer a plan of action and hope.

Motivate

- Help the patient to appreciate the disadvantages of abuse and the advantages of sobriety.
- Say that you know that it is difficult but possible.
- Convey the concept of shared responsibility.

Action

If there is a history of withdrawal symptoms or withdrawal convulsions, admit the patient to a local hospital and detoxify.

Detoxification

Hospitalize the patient. Administer diazepam 5–10 mg orally every three to six hours (the worst withdrawal symptoms occur in the first forty-eight hours and the patient may need high doses of diazepam). If the patient is in alcohol withdrawal delirium and is very restless, lorazepam 2–4 mg intramuscularly (IM) may be administered when needed. The diazepam must be discontinued over five to fourteen days as the withdrawal symptoms subside. As an alternative to diazepam, carbamazepine 200–600 mg per day may be administered. This is not an established treatment at present.

Proper physical work-up is essential. Infection, bleeding from the gastro-intestinal tract, trauma, malnutrition, and metabolic disorders are common. Most alcoholics in withdrawal are not dehydrated and over-hydration must be avoided.

Thiamine (Vitamin B1) 100 mg must be administered IMI or orally for seven days. If the patient is on a glucose drip the thiamine should be administered with the intravenous infusion. A multivitamin supplement should also be prescribed. Once the patient has resumed a healthy diet, this supplement may be discontinued after two weeks.

Place the patient in a safe environment and monitor intake and output during the period of hospitalization. An alcoholic in withdrawal might be restless because of autonomic over-activity and hallucinations. Anxious caretakers must avoid over-sedation. If sedation is sufficient, no anticonvulsant need be prescribed. If a withdrawal seizure occurs, intravenous diazepam 5–20 mg may be needed.

After detoxification, the patient should be encouraged to enter a suitable programme. The use of disulfiram should be discussed. The patient should be informed of the danger of using alcohol after taking disulfiram, and should take disulfiram voluntarily. On taking alcohol with disulfiram, the first metabolite of alcohol, acetaldehyde, accumulates in the blood and the patient becomes flushed, nauseated, and dizzy, with malaise and palpitations for thirty to sixty minutes. Disulfiram should not be started within twenty-four hours of having consumed alcohol. Its effect may last as long as two weeks. Disulfiram may motivate the patient to avoid alcohol during stressful periods.

Even after a successfully completed programme, the primary therapist should maintain contact with the patient.

Alcohol-induced psychiatric disorders

Alcohol hallucinosis

This condition usually manifests as auditory hallucinations without obvious signs of withdrawal delirium, but may occur in intoxication or in withdrawal. The patient may become extremely frightened and restless, and pose a serious suicide risk. Admit the patient, sedate if restless (lorazepam 2–4 mg IMI), and start haloperidol 5–10 mg, either IMI or orally, two to three times a day. Haloperidol may be discontinued two to four weeks after all symptoms have subsided. The patient should not take alcohol again, as even small amounts may trigger the hallucinations.

Alcohol dementia

Even young patients may develop signs of dementia, for instance personality deterioration, personal neglect, and memory failure. Some of these changes are reversible if the patient can maintain sobriety.

Alcohol amnesic disorder

After an episode of acute thiamine deficiency (ataxia, delirium, nystagmus, and cranial nerve III, IV, and VI opthalmoplegia), an individual may develop a permanent inability to store new information. Patients may fill the gaps with untruths (confabulation). Thiamine supplementation is of the utmost importance in avoiding this disorder.

Alcohol-related mood, anxiety, sleep, and sexual disorders are only reversible once alcohol intake has been stopped.

Note: Alcoholism can be treated. Be energetic, persistent, and kind but firm.

Cannabis

Street names for cannabis include dagga, grass, pot, joints, ganja, and tea. Experimentation is common among children and adolescents. Only a small percentage will become regular users and even fewer will become abusers. It is called a 'gateway drug' because it may open the door to other drugs and the 'drugging' subculture. A small percentage of adults claim that cannabis can be used socially without any detrimental effects.

Cannabis sativa is the plant of origin, and tetrahydrocannabinol the psychoactive substance.

Intoxication

Cannabis may produce euphoria, anxiety, a sensation of slowed time, impaired motor coordination, and maladaptive behaviour or social withdrawal. There may be increased appetite, conjunctival injection, dry mouth, and tachycardia.

Dependence

Mild withdrawal symptoms such as irritability, restlessness, insomnia, anorexia, and mild nausea may develop. Diazepam 5–15 mg per day for five to ten days may be helpful.

Cannabis-induced psychosis

This condition is discussed in the section on substance-induced psychosis.

Cannabis amotivational syndrome

This condition is associated with chronic heavy cannabis abuse and is characterized by unwillingness to persist at tasks, and by anergia and apathy.

Treatment

The patient must be treated according to the basic principles applied to substance abuse patients as previously discussed. Cannabis may be detected in the urine up to four weeks after last use.

Methaqualone

Street names for the drug are Mandrax, buttons, and sproeitjies. This is a non-barbiturate sedative-hypnotic, and is usually smoked, often with cannabis.

Intoxication

Intoxication is accompanied by dry mouth, headache, dizziness, diarrhoea, chills, tremors, paraesthesia, epistaxis, and urticaria.

Overdose

Overdose results in restlessness, delirium, muscle spasms, convulsions, and death.

Dependence

Users develop tolerance for this drug. Withdrawal symptoms are headaches, muscle spasms, and convulsions.

Detoxification

Benzodiazepines are the drugs indicated during detoxification.

Amphetamine-like drugs (stimulants)

These include:
- dextroamphetamine (Dexedrine);

- methylphenidate (Ritalin);
- ecstacy (E Raves, Love doves, Adams etc.);
- ephedrine (Speed); and
- appetite suppressants.

Intoxication

Intoxication is accompanied by euphoria or blunted affect, hypervigilance, pupil dilatation, sweatiness and chills, weight loss, anger, and psychomotor agitation or retardation.

Withdrawal (crash)

Withdrawal symptoms include fatigue, unpleasant dreams, depressed mood, insomnia or hypersomnia, increased appetite, withdrawal or agitation, muscle and stomach cramps, and profuse sweating.

Detoxification

Short-term benzodiazepines are presecribed for severe anxiety. If severe ongoing depression is present, antidepressants should be considered.

Cocaine-related disorders

Street names for cocaine include crack, coke, and snow. This is the most addictive of abused substances.

Intoxication

Intoxication is characterized by elation, heightened self-esteem, and subjective judgement on improvement of mental and physical tasks. High doses of cocaine are associated with agitation, impaired judgement, and restlessness. Physical symptoms are tachycardia, hypertension, and mydriasis.

Withdrawal

Withdrawal is accompanied by depression (crash), anxiety, irritability, fatigue, and hypersomnia.

Detoxification

Detoxification can be achieved with the aid of admission, support, and short-term benzodiazepines.

Hallucinogen-related disorders

Psychedelics or psychotomimetics in the form of LSD go by the street names caps, trips, microdots, and candy.

Intoxication

Intoxication is characterized by a fear of losing one's mind, paranoid ideation, intensification of sensations, derealization, and hallucinations. Physical symptoms are pupillary dilatation, tachycardia, sweating, tremor, and lack of coordination. Hallucinogens may cause *flashbacks* of the symptoms experienced during intoxication.

Withdrawal

There are no withdrawal symptoms associated with hallucinogen use.

Treatment

The preferred treatment for intoxication is 'talking the patient down'. Support the patient and reassure him or her that the symptoms are drug induced and temporary. With severe intoxication, haloperidol 5–10 mg IMI or lorazepam 2–4 mg IMI may be needed to calm the patient down.

Inhalant-related disorders

These disorders result from inhalation of petrol, thinners, 'rubber cement', Tippex thinners, glue, and spray-paint aerosols.

Intoxication

Intoxication is characterized by initial stimulation, euphoria, and a floating effect, which may be followed by fearfulness, hallucinations, and eventual suppression of perception, affect, and responsiveness. Physical symptoms include slurred speech, ataxia, lethargy, depressed reflexes, double vision, and muscle weakness. Serious intoxication may result in respiratory depression, arrhythmias, coma, and death. Avoid the use of benzodiazepines for sedation during intoxication as respiratory arrest may follow. If sedation is needed, use haloperidol 5–10 mg IM.

Withdrawal

Withdrawal symptoms are rare.

Opioid-related disorders

Painkillers are the most common opioids and include wellconal (pinks), heroin (smack), and codeine-containing medication (Phensidyl).

Intoxication

Intoxication is accompanied by initial euphoria followed by apathy, and psychomotor agitation or retardation. Physical symptoms are pupillary constriction, slurred speech, and impaired attention and memory.

Withdrawal

Symptoms of withdrawal include intense craving, dysphoric mood, muscle aches, lacrimation, rhinorrhea, pupillary dilatation, sweating, yawning, fever, and insomnia.

Detoxification

The patient must be admitted. Observation and benzodiazepines are prescribed for mild withdrawal. For severe heroin withdrawal, methadone 20–80 mg a day may be administered. Methadone causes dependence and should be withdrawn as soon as patients stabilize. Clonidine 0.1–0.3 mg three to four times a day may also be administered during opioid withdrawal.

Phencyclidine-related disorders

The relevant substances are PCP, angel-dust, crystal, peace, and so forth.

Intoxication

Abusers become agitated, assaultive, unpredictable, impulsive, hallucinated, disorientated, and confused. Nystagmus, tachycardia, hypertension, ataxia, muscle rigidity, and seizures may occur during intoxication. Autonomic instability and hypothermia, renal failure, and hypertension may cause death. Urgent benzodiazepine treatment may be needed during intoxication.

Long-term abusers may suffer memory loss, dull thinking, depression, lethargy, and impaired concentration.

Withdrawal

There is no physical withdrawal syndrome.

Treatment

Treatment involves admission and management of physical complications. Neuroleptics should be avoided.

Sedative-, hypnotic-, or anxiolytic-related disorders

Benzodiazepines are the causative substances of these disorders.

Intoxication

Sedation, slurred speech, unsteady gait, and impaired attention and memory are symptoms. These disorders may also be associated with behavioural disinhibition (hostile, aggressive), lability, and impaired judgement.

Withdrawal

Anxiety, dysphoria, nausea, sweating, restlessness, and convulsions are symptoms associated with withdrawal.

Detoxification

Patient co-operation is an essential element in this process. If withdrawal symptoms are severe the patient must be admitted. Dosage must be reduced gradually over weeks and months.

Substance-induced psychiatric disorders other than intoxication and withdrawal

- Acute and chronic use and abuse of substances may induce psychotic, mood, anxiety, sexual, and sleep disorders.
- These disorders are not merely the effects of intoxication and withdrawal. They may well be triggered by intoxication and withdrawal but will still be present even after the actual intoxication and withdrawal symptoms have subsided.
- They do not usually persist for longer than a month after the cessation of substance use.
- They do not always reverse after cessation of the drug.
- They do not have the typical onset, phenomenology, and course of the non-substance-induced psychotic, mood, anxiety, sexual, and sleep disorders.
- Substance-induced psychotic disorders should be treated with antipsychotic drugs for between two and four weeks after the last psychotic symptoms.
- A serious and ongoing mood disorder should be treated as a major depressive episode on therapeutic doses of antidepressants for at least six months.
- Anxiety disorders and substance abuse may be co-morbid disorders. After substance withdrawal, the anxiety symptoms should be re-evaluated and followed by diagnosis and appropriate treatment.
- Sleep disorders may persist for a while but should reverse without hypnotics. Most hypnotics are habit-forming and should be avoided by addicts where possible.

22 HIV/Aids

Aids has become the world's most serious public health problem. In South-Africa, Aids has reached epidemic levels, and as most of the problems associated with HIV infection can be dealt with at primary health care level, it is crucial that nurses be able to counsel, support, and care for people who are ill and dying, and that they educate communities on prevention strategies to control the spread of HIV.

HIV infection and Aids has an enormous physical, emotional, psychological, and social impact. It puts tremendous pressure on relationships, families, and the broader community.

Infected people, their partners, families, and close friends therefore often need support during this difficult time and caring for people with HIV/Aids calls for both medical and psychosocial support.

In the primary health care situation nurses will find that counselling and care of people with HIV/Aids is an increasing component of their work. The focus of this chapter will be on meeting the counselling needs of HIV-positive patients, supporting their families, and educating the wider community.

Principles of counselling

The following principles are important when counselling patients with HIV/Aids (they also apply to other counselling contexts):

- *Confidentiality:* HIV/Aids patients have the right to confidentiality and professionalism.
- *Respect:* Nurses should respect their patient's confidences and decisions so that patients learn to trust and confide.
- *Unconditional acceptance:* A non-judgemental, accepting approach allows patients to be open about their feelings and concerns. HIV/Aids patients may experience discrimination and this acceptance is therefore particularly important.
- *Professionalism:* The counselling relationship is not a friendship. Where friends may become over-involved in a patient's problems, counsellors should maintain a controlled relationship with patients that provides a more balanced approach.
- *Empathy:* It is crucial that nurses be able to empathize with patients and really try to understand the pain that they're experiencing.

Pre-test counselling

The HIV test can raise many issues and fears. Patients will need to discuss these both before and after the test. Before an HIV test nurses should:

- Explain the purpose of the test. Patients should also know what the results will mean. A positive result, for instance, does not mean that the person has Aids yet. A first negative test may fall in the 'window' period that occurs after early infection, when the test does not detect the virus. The 'window' period is between three to six months. If the person has been raped, suffered a needle-stick injury, or had positive sexual contact, the test should be repeated.
- Inform the patient about the test, i.e. what to expect and how long it will take. Inform patients that the test takes

fewer than five minutes, and is not painful. They should understand that if the first test is positive, a second test will be done on the same blood sample using a different kit, and that two positive tests indicate a conclusive positive test result.

- Determine whether the patient is at risk, i.e. has had positive sexual contact, a positive needle-stick injury, or received a blood transfusion with possible infected blood.
- Ensure that the patient understands the implications of the test and educate the patient about how a positive test would impact on his or her life. A positive test will not mean that the patient is dying, and in most cases the patient will only develop Aids within seven to ten years from the time of infection.
- Prepare the patient for a possible positive result.
- Educate the patient about future prevention, i.e. using a condom, limiting sexual partners, and not sharing needles.

Post-test counselling

Informing HIV-negative patients

- Patients should be informed as soon as possible. Avoid delay.
- Always provide results in a private and confidential manner, as the patient may be anxious and fearful.
- Make sure patients understand the meaning and implications of a negative test, and the need for a second test, where necessary.
- Educate patients about continued prevention.

Informing HIV-positive patients

Dealing with the patient's reaction

Make sure that you are in a quiet and private place where you cannot be interrupted. Don't rush the session. Acknowledge the patient's feelings. Remember to allow and encourage the patient to express feelings. Crying, sobbing, and angry outbursts are ways that people unburden themselves. Remember that not all problems are solvable but that just talking about the problem and sharing fears, worries, and concerns, helps the patient to cope. Always provide patients with the opportunity for follow-up.

Informing the family

Discuss how to inform the family. The decision to inform the family is always the patient's. People often worry about how their families will react when they tell them that they are HIV-positive. However, patients should understand that they have a moral obligation to inform their sexual partners, and to prevent the spread of Aids.

Avoid giving too much advice. The patient must still maintain responsibility for decisions or actions.

Discussing health and sexuality issues

Discuss the changes that will have to be made to the patient's health and sexual practices.

Discussing pregnancy

Pregnancy raises many questions for HIV-positive individuals. Affected people need to start making important decisions about whether to have another child or not, and sometimes whether to terminate a pregnancy.

If the patient is pregnant, discuss the risk to the mother and to the newborn baby. It is often uncertain whether the baby is HIV-positive and parents need to know that it may take up to eighteen months to finally find this out.

Dealing with patients at risk

Assess patients for risk of suicide.

Offering support

Offer ongoing counselling support to the family and the patient. Show your support for the patient's decisions and always make sure that patients feel free to return for follow-up or further counselling.

Discussing medical intervention

Educate patients about the medical treatments available. Prepare them for what to expect.

Counselling HIV-positive patients

Denial

People with HIV infection often have great difficulty believing or accepting that they have a serious condition. This often results in people not returning to follow-up or continuing with unsafe sexual practices.

Counselling may be difficult if there is denial. However, it is very important in helping a patient accept his or her HIV infection. Counselling will help the patient develop a responsible and positive attitude.

Living with uncertainty

People with HIV/Aids may have many unanswered questions:

- 'Where did I get the infection from?'
- 'Can I become ill and when will it happen?'
- 'Can I pass it on to my children?'
- 'Will there be any treatment for me?'
- 'Will I die?'
- 'How will people react?'

Living with these uncertainties can be a tremendous burden and the nurse can help by listening carefully (responsive listening); acknowledging the patient's feelings and putting them in context; clarifying the message ('So you're saying that the main problem is your fear of dying?'); remembering to use open-ended questioning techniques; summarizing periodically; observing body language; showing interest and support; and perhaps even constructing a short-term plan of action for follow-up sessions.

Relationships

HIV and Aids can severely strain relationships with loved ones, families, and friends. Your patients may need to talk about whether to disclose their HIV-positive status. They may also want to know how to tell people. HIV-positive individuals often fear rejection or blame from their partners and they may have feelings of guilt and shame. Re-establishing trust after disclosure may be important.

Support systems

Determine what kind of support systems the patient and family have in place.

Coping with illness

The counsellor needs to support patients (and often their loved ones as well) through repeated illnesses and deterioration in health. You may have to help your patients look at ways of living each day, rather than thinking too far ahead into the future. You may have to explore ways of making the quality rather than the quantity of life better.

Suicide and depression

Counselling is often required to help deal with the feelings of rejection, guilt, and blame. It is also important to note that the uncertainty patients often experience may lead to depression and risk of suicide

Discrimination

People affected by HIV and Aids are often subjected to discrimination and rejection by their friends, work colleagues, insurance schemes, and even families and partners. Support and counselling and even legal advice may be needed. Coping with unemployment may be an issue.

Sexuality

Being HIV-positive means having to make major changes to one's sexual behaviour and/or the way one has sex. This, in itself, can be extremely difficult and can stress relationships with lovers and partners.

HIV infection may also mean having to come to terms with, and be open about, homosexuality. This may be a difficult and trying process.

Coping with losses

People with HIV suffer many losses. They lose their health, their independence, and many years of life. They may also lose their lover or spouse, their job, their financial security, and their usual life and lifestyle. They need to change their sexual habits. Many pregnancies end in termination or abortion. Parents may need help coping with an HIV-infected newborn and may also experience feelings of guilt and anger if their infant is HIV-positive or when their infant becomes ill or dies. It is important to counsel patients and help them cope with loss. Counselling may be useful for all members of the family, such as children, grandparents, lovers, and friends, as loss of a loved one has an extended influence.

Referring patients

With all the above-mentioned problems, people suffering from HIV or Aids often feel overwhelmed and despondent. They feel their problems are too big, too new, too much. In this way, counselling can be very helpful.

Nurses can provide counselling, without becoming over-involved in patients' personal lives. The counsellor can offer help that is fair, professional, and balanced.

A counsellor can often help calm and stabilize people during crises. Finally, Aids can cause much shame, guilt, and embarrassment. Counselling can help a patient to handle these feelings, and to face the world with confidence and dignity again.

Counselling is a process that helps people understand and deal with their problems and communicate better with those with whom they are emotionally involved. The counsellor discusses and explores the feelings, worries, and concerns of the patient. Together they look at ways of dealing and coping with these feelings and concerns as well as possible.

Counselling does not involve merely giving advice. It also does not mean taking over the patient's problem. It means encouraging them to find their own solutions to problems, which helps them to become confident and independent again.

Nurses may find that they are not coping with a patient or

that the issues and problems are too complex and difficult. They may need to refer such patients to a more experienced counsellor or to someone who has more time for counselling. If necessary, patients could be referred to a clinical psychologist in their area. The primary health care nurse should have an updated referral list for this purpose.

Educating the community

Nurses can assist in creating Aids awareness by undertaking psychoeducation within the community. They can also conduct awareness campaigns, and initiate programmes in the clinics. For example, they can distribute free condoms in clinics.

23 Epilepsy

A seizure results from a sudden electrical discharge of cerebral neurones. If the discharge or burst comes from only one part of the brain this is a focal or partial seizure; if the whole brain (i.e. both sides) discharges simultaneously a generalized seizure results. A single seizure, for example in a diabetic with low sugar, is not uncommon. More than one seizure would indicate epilepsy.

The cause

In many patients there will not appear to be a cause for epilepsy. The cause may be genetic or familial and no cause can be identified, even with the most sophisticated tests. However, the patient should always be questioned and examined for a precipitating cause. Removal of such a cause may prevent epileptic fits.

Causes to exclude are:
- head injuries;

- infections such as meningitis or encephalitis (acute infections) or more chronic infections such as cysticercosis or Aids;
- alcohol;
- underlying tumors or vascular disease; and
- birth injuries.

New injuries or infections, hormonal changes, sleep deprivation, use of, or sudden withdrawal from, alcohol or drugs, dehydration, or malnutrition may bring on seizures in a patient who is known to be subject to epileptic seizures.

Age of onset and biological history

Epilepsy can develop at any age and in both sexes. Newborn babies can have fits from birth injuries, an aged person can have a fit after a stroke or a head injury. Between 2 and 5 per cent of the population may experience a seizure, that is one in twenty people; and 0,5 per cent, (one in 200) will be left with chronic epilepsy. In 60 to 70 per cent of patients with epilepsy it may not be possible to find a cause. Approximately 70 to 80 per cent of epileptics will show a natural remission over a period of fifteen to twenty years. About 20 per cent of all epileptics will be extremely difficult to control. In the untreated state about a third of patients have less than one attack a year, a third have between one and twelve seizures a year and a third may have more than one seizure a month, sometimes even one a week.

Nevertheless, approximately 60 to 70 per cent of all epileptic patients will be well controlled by using monotherapy, namely one drug at proper therapeutic levels (calculated by dose per kg of body weight). Because epilepsy is a problem in 30 per cent of patients and is easy to control in 70 per cent of patients, the vast majority of epileptic patients can be successfully treated in clinics and community hospitals. In fact, the problems in most epileptic patients relate less to the actual seizure and more to psychosocial and employment issues.

Clinical history

The patient's symptoms and complaints form the basis of the clinical presentations. The symptoms and signs reported by family and friends may be equally important.

It is frequently difficult to be sure that the patient is in fact describing an epileptic fit. A surprising number of doctors, nurses, and medical students have never seen a convulsion. A patient who has a fit in the clinic or hospital is hence often treated as an emergency, yet when the same fit occurs at home the family will cope adequately. Where any form of 'blackout' has occurred, both the patient and someone who has witnessed the event must be questioned. Remember that the patient may have been unconscious and afterwards confused and have no real recollection of the attack. Table 23.1 lists a useful set of questions to be put to the patient. Table 23.2 lists the questions for the witness or family member. This may provide assistance in deciding whether the blackout was in fact a seizure, and a good description may help to localize the site of origin of the epileptogenic lesion.

Table 23.1 Questions for the patient

- What were you doing before the attack?
- What was the first thing you noticed that seemed to be abnormal?
- What happened after that until you lost your consciousness?
- Were you fully unconscious, in other words, was there a period where you were totally unaware of your environment?
- What is the first thing you remember after having regained consciousness?
- Were you confused?
- Did you lose control of your bladder?
- Did you bite your tongue?
- Were you tired and did you go to sleep?
- Did your muscles ache afterwards?

Table 23.2 Questions for the family

- Was the patient unconscious (i.e. lack of responsiveness)?
- What was the patient's position when the attack occurred?
- Was the patient able to control the seizure?
- Was this a single episode or a series?
- Did the patient recover between attacks?
- What was the patient's colour?
- Ask all the 'patient's' questions and check the events before and after the seizure against the questions in Table 23.1.
- What did the patient look like during the event – for example rigid, jerking, teeth clenched?
- What medication does the patient use?

The purpose of the history is to find out not only whether the event was a seizure but also what type of seizure it was. Treatment efficacy is influenced by seizure type. Tables 23.3 and 23.4 classify seizure types into generalized and partial seizures. With some practice it becomes fairly easy to determine the difference between the two groups.

Table 23.3 Classification of partial epileptic seizures

A Simple partial (consciousness not impaired)
- With motor signs, namely march (Jacksonian), postural, phonatory.
- With somatosensory or special sensory symptoms (light flashes, somatosensory, visual, auditory, olfactory, gustatory, vertiginous).
- With autonomic symptoms or signs (epigastric sensation, pallor, sweating, flushing, pilo-erection, pupillary dilation).
- With psychic symptoms (very rare – usually part of complex partial seizures).

B Complex partial seizures
- Beginning as simple partial seizures and progressing to impairment of consciousness:
  - With no other features;

Table 23.3 continued

- With features as in A above; and/or
- With automatisms.
- Unconscious from the onset with similar features to rest of B above.

C Partial seizures evolving to generalized tonic-clonic convulsions (secondary generalized)

Table 23.4 Classification of generalized epileptic seizures

A Typical absences
B Myoclonic seizures – single or multiple
C Tonic seizures
D Tonic-clonic seizures
E Atonic seizures

Classification of absense seizures

- Impaired consciousness only.
- With mild clonic component.
- With atonic component.
- With automatisms.
- With autonomic components.

Note: Combinations of the above types may occur

Partial seizures

Simple partial seizures, for example Jacksonian seizures, are epileptic seizures that may originate in any one part of the brain except the temporal lobe, and remain localized without spread and with no loss of consciousness. Partial seizures that remain localized in the temporal lobe usually alter consciousness because the limbic system of the brain is in the temporal lobe. These are known as complex partial seizures or temporal lobe epilepsy (TLE). As up to 70 per cent of all seizures, especially TLE seizures, fit into the partial category, it is important to define the group carefully. The commonest presentation of this group of seizures is the one that is best known to most medical personnel. The seizure starts in one part of the brain and then generalizes to involve the whole brain.

The patient has an aura, which progresses to a generalized tonic clonic seizure. During the seizure:

- there is total spasm of all muscles in the body;
- the patient goes blue because respiration is not working;
- the tongue is bitten because the jaw clamps shut;
- the oesophagus is in spasm and saliva drools from the mouth because the patient cannot swallow;
- the patient experiences incontinence of bladder and even bowel owing to the intense contraction of the bladder and bowel muscles;
- all muscles are in tight spasm and feel very tired and may even ache after the attack; and
- after the attack the patient is usually confused and wants to sleep.

Apart from the description of the attack from a witness, the most important part of this history is the description of the aura, i.e. what was the first thing the patient noted as being abnormal before losing consciousness? The description of the aura will help determine the anatomical origin of the seizure in the brain.

If the aura was one of the special senses, for example a peculiar smell, taste, or sound, the fit started in the temporal lobe. If the aura was a jerking of the face or hand, the fit started in the motor area of the brain.

Patients with complex partial seizures or temporal lobe epilepsy are sometimes misdiagnosed as hysteria because they may present with other symptoms or signs that look very bizarre. The reason is that the temporal lobe controls memory and emotion. These patients may thus behave aggressively or may recognize a place they have never actually seen before (dèja vú). Temporal lobe epilepsy patients have different attacks on different occasions.

They may sometimes just have a momentary loss of consciousness (absence), while on other occasions they may have repetitive movements such as lip smacking (automatisms) and sometimes a full blown tonic-clonic seizure as described above.

Generalized seizures

These patients have no aura. The reason is that the fit does not start in either a lobe or one hemisphere but engulfs the whole brain immediately. The patient always loses consciousness but may recover very quickly. The most common types of generalized seizures are absences and tonic-clonic seizures.

Previously these attacks used to be called petit mal and grand mal. However, as treatment depends on defining whether the seizure is partial or generalized it is clinically much more helpful to describe the attack as:

- with or without aura;
- with or without loss of consciousness;
- with or without tonic and/or clonic movements; and
- with or without post-ictal confusion.

Less common general seizures may be:

- tonic (spasm only);
- clonic (jerking only);
- atonic (complete loss of tone); or
- myoclonic (intermittent brief generalized jerks).

Clinical examination

The purpose of the examination is to establish whether the patient is still manifesting features of an attack and if there are any focal or precipitating signs.

First establish the mental state. If this is abnormal, establish whether this is a recent or established situation. Many epileptic patients are mentally challenged from birth. If the abnormality is recent determine the cause, for example:

- post-ictal confusion or drowsiness (part of the attack);

- pyrexia;
- neck stiffness (the cause may be meningitis);
- flushed and history of alcohol (alcohol withdrawal).

Check routine medical signs. Exclude diabetic coma, hypoglycaemia, hypotension, dehydration, cardiac arrhythmias, anoxia, and respiratory failure. If any of these are present, treatment may stop the fits.

Is the patient in status epilepticus, in other words, does the patient recover consciousness before the next fit occurs? A patient in status epilepticus will die unless treated rapidly and, if necessary, ventilated and hospitalized as soon as possible.

Now examine the patient for focal neurological signs, for example unequal pupils, unilateral weakness, cranial nerve palsies, and papilloedema.

Medical treatment

Pharmacological management is the cornerstone of therapy (see Table 23.5) and is successful in 70 per cent of patients. Use monotherapy, one drug at a time to full dosage. Only if a patient cannot be controlled with monotherapy or if a focal or reversible secondary cause is suspected should the patient be referred to a secondary care regional hospital. Since the nurse is responsible for maintaining the medication, a basic knowledge of the medication and its side-effects, is valuable.

Table 23.5 Pharmacokinetic and therapeutic data

Drug family	Daily dose	Half-life	Prominence of side effects	Type of epilepsy
Hydantoins				
Phenytoin	5–7 mg/kg	24 hrs	Moderate	Generalized or complex partial

Table 23.5 continued

Carbamazepine	10–30 mg/kg	12 hrs	Moderate	Partial seizures or generalized
Benzodiazepines				
Diazepam	0,5 mg/kg	30 hrs	High	Absences or generalized (Myoclonic/atonic)
Clonazepam	0,1–0,2 mg/kg	30 hrs	High	
Succinimides				
Ethosuximide	20–30 mg/kg	40 hrs	Low	Absences
Barbiturates				
Phenobarbitone	3–8 mg/kg	96 hrs	High	Major generalized
Valproate				
Valproic acid	20–30 mg/kg	8 hrs	Low	Absences or generalized or partial seizures

However, all anti-epileptic drugs have side-effects that may be idiosyncratic and can be caused by excessive dosage. These drugs may result in non-compliance, which will often be diminished if therapy is introduced gradually. Drowsiness, impaired cognition, and cerebellar ataxia are the commonest effects of overdose. Bone-marrow depression, hepatotoxicity, and severe skin reactions occur as idiosyncratic reactions. Women who are trying to fall pregnant should be pretreated with folic acid to prevent neural tube defects; but if an epileptic who is on therapy is already pregnant there is no point in changing medication. The newer anti-epileptic drugs should not be initiated in a primary care setting. If a patient requires these drugs for control it should be under the guidance of a neurologist or physician in a secondary or tertiary care facility. Routine drug level monitoring is never required in fit-free, compliant patients. The basic rules of management of an epileptic patient are out lined in Table 23.6.

When to refer to a secondary hospital

Refer to a secondary hospital in any of the situations mentioned below.

- If there are more than twelve attacks a year and they cannot be controlled by monotherapy.
- Where a case of status epilepticus is not responding to diazepam and phenytoin, IV therapy must be initiated urgently. A knowledgeable member of staff must accompany the patient. Make sure that a drip is set up and that the patient is intubated so that respiratory resuscitation can be started immediately.
- If there are unexplained focal signs or papilloedema.
- If a secondary cause, for example bradyarrhythmia, cannot be treated successfully.

Table 23.6 Management of epilepsy

- Identify type of epilepsy.
- Do not treat first seizure unless focal signs or a cause is found.
- Do not treat intermittently.
- Continue treatment for two years after last seizure.
- Use monotherapy to therapeutic levels.
- Use minimum number of drugs.
- Test serum levels if control or compliance is poor.
- Do not allow any epileptic to drive public or commercial vehicles.
- An epileptic may drive private vehicles if seizure-free for two years.
- Introduce therapy slowly and increase dosage over two weeks to minimize side-effects.

Nursing management

- Epilepsy is a *chronic illness*; it therefore needs adjustment, not cure. Adjustment involves successfully negotiating a change in self-image to accommodate this new aspect. These patients often need therapy to cope with change.
- To be able to adjust, epileptic patients need effective coping strategies. People with epilepsy tend to view themselves and their condition as unacceptable and are thus less likely to seek support. This is due to negative attitudes towards people with epilepsy and prejudiced attitudes in the area of employment.
- Family psychoeducation fosters acceptance of the epileptic family member and reduces stigma.
- Explore the person's belief system about self and about the condition and its implications for his or her life-style. Provide psychoeducation about the condition, the medication and its effects, the precipitating factors, and injury precautions, to correct beliefs based on lack of knowledge.
- Assist the person to understand that beliefs influence the way he or she thinks and behaves. Ask the person to match the beliefs with the identified situations and then, next to each pair, list the ways he or she behaves and the feelings he or she has in each situation.
- Help patients focus on situations in which they feel competent, as this will enhance self-image and coping skills.
- Examine and explore positive and negative consequences of the coping responses.
- Develop effective coping behaviours. Patients must engage actively in the problem-solving process since the aim is to facilitate a sense of mastery and control.
- When people in control of their lives, life has meaning and they can cope with the fact that epilepsy is a chronic, life-long disease.

Traditionally too much emphasis has been placed on an individual's seizures and deficiencies rather than on strengths, abilities, and overall capacity. This approach needs to be remedied, if the person is to negotiate a successful change in self-image and is to accommodate epilepsy as only one aspect of himself of herself.

24 Rehabilitation of chronic patients

Psychiatric illness can be devastating and the adverse effects are often worse than those of physical illness such as coronary artery disease or arthritis (Uys, 1997). The seriousness of this impairment, and the fact that patients are at home for the greatest part of their illness, creates an extra burden for the family – it can dominate the lives of family members and destroy family relations.

Intensive efforts are therefore necessary to rehabilitate these patients. In South Africa, psychiatric community services are still fragmented and in the deinstitutional era – the focus must still shift from treatment to rehabilitation. In the current context, the focus is still very much on diagnosis and treatment, and not on rehabilitation.

Certain aspects of rehabilitation have received some attention, namely vocational rehabilitation and alternative housing. In terms of vocational rehabilitation, there is limited access to sheltered employment workshops. More creative options are generally not available.

Nurses should play a crucial role in the rehabilitation of psychiatric patients with chronic illness. This will enable them to provide follow-up care and maintain stable chronic patients within the community.

Psychosocial rehabilitation

Psychosocial rehabilitation is a process that aims to improve the functioning of psychiatric patients within a specific environment, i.e. within their own family and in the community.

Elements of psychosocial rehabilitation

The basic elements of rehabilitation interventions are:

- *Increasing skills:* This refers to improving general life skills or specific vocational skills, either in the patient or the family. An increase in skills assists the whole network to cope better with stress, and, in some instances it can prevent stress.
- *Increasing support:* Any action that can increase the support that the patient and family receive assists in preventing breakdown and promoting health. This refers to entitlements (disability grants), material assistance, and psychosocial support.
- *Manipulating resources:* This may include aspects such as marketing the patient to a service, or marketing a service to a patient. But it might need to go further in negotiating changes in the service to make it more appropriate to the patient. It might also mean advocating service improvement or service creation.
- *Optimizing symptom control:* The successful rehabilitation of the patient depends on optimal symptom control. This is usually done through medication, although psychotherapy may play a role. Medication to control symptoms may be adequate for staying at home, but not for working. Therefore, the rehabilitation worker needs to work closely with the person treating the patient.
- *General public education:* Reintegration of the patient into society depends on the attitude of the general public, and also on specific groups, such as employers. Changes in attitudes need to be addressed purposefully and specifically, and this articulates closely with increasing support for patients and their families, i.e. the stigma that the public attaches to people with mental illness needs to change.

Community services in South Africa generally have very few of the available rehabilitation technologies in place. The major technologies that have developed in this field or have been incorporated into it, are listed below. These technologies form the basic building blocks of a community-based rehabilitation programme. They combine the basic elements of rehabilitation to address the needs of the patient, often in a specific area of living.

- *Psychoeducation*: This refers to the process where patients and their families are taught about the treatment and management of mental illness so that they can cope better with community-based care. Currently patients and their families have very little information, and often not even a diagnosis. Vague terms such as 'nervous breakdown' are still used frequently. Psychoeducation is an intensive and responsive teaching process. It empowers the family and the patient with knowledge and skills, and can make a dramatic difference to the long-term outcome for patients.

- *Case management*: This is an approach to long-term care that addresses all the needs of disabled people. It aims to assess their needs, link them to a variety of services, and coordinate service use to achieve a successful outcome. Although there are different models of case management, the generalist model seems to be most appropriate for the South African situation. In this model; one person, who may belong to any of the helping professions, deals with the problems of the patient without keeping strictly to professional boundaries (Uys, 1995). It gives the consumer an identifiable, consistent helper in the complex health system.

- *Skills teaching*: This is the structured teaching of the deficient life skills needed in the specific social, vocational, and living environment of the disabled person. This can be done during day programmes or group sessions.

- *Vocational rehabilitation*: This process enables the disabled person to secure, retain, and advance in suitable employment. The aim is integrated and competitive employment. This means that the person works for at least minimum wages or better, with non-disabled co-workers, at a job that provides room for advancement in settings that produce valued goods and services. The favoured way of achieving this is through Supported Employment (SE).

- *Appropriate housing:* The housing of disabled people should suit their own needs and life-styles and optimize social and vocational functioning. This involves a range of housing options, from group homes to single accommodation.

Functional assessment

Patients who live with a chronic mental illness often have functional deficits that remain even if they are well. In many situations, not enough attention is given to these areas of poor functioning, which can have a negative impact on patients. Functioning is often the area of greatest difficulty for patients as it affects their ability to perform everyday tasks.

If you have a patient who is not able to carry out routine tasks, it is essential to refer that person to an occupational therapist (OT) for a functional assessment. After the functional assessment the OT will suggest strategies that aim to maximize the potential of the patient. The strategies also assist patients to become as independent as possible.

If there is no occupational therapist working in your region, here are some issues to consider when assessing whether a patient has suffered a decline in functioning.

When assessing a patient's functional ability consider the following four areas:

- *Personal management:* This includes the ability of patients to look after themselves and their belongings, as well as to perform tasks that are expected of them around the home, such as cooking, cleaning, gardening, caring for children, and budgeting. Also consider their ability to get from one place to another.
- *Social functioning:* This includes the patient's ability to interact appropriately and consistently with people in his or her environment, both familiar and unfamiliar. It also includes their ability to initiate and maintain

conversations, as well as to handle conflict and avoid situations in which they feel uncomfortable.

- *Work:* This area involves the ability to perform tasks. The tasks might be part of a job or they may be tasks in the home that are equivalent to a job, such as looking after children or doing housework. They should be able to be punctual, to behave appropriately, and to work through a task at an acceptable rate and quality.
- *Leisure:* This includes the patient's ability to use free time constructively and to be able to understand the importance of having free time.

When screening for the level of a patient's functional ability, there are other questions that patients or relatives will need to answer. The answers to these questions indicate levels of independence in each area of a patient's life.

- Is the patient able to perform tasks independently or is constant support and encouragement needed?
- Is the person able to initiate a task or are they only able to complete a task that has been initiated for them?
- Does the person behave appropriately?
- Does the person accept constructive feedback and can she or he integrate feedback and improve?
- Is the person's behaviour consistent?
- Is the person able to work at an acceptable rate?
- Is the quality of the performance adequate?
- Is the person able to evaluate his or her own performance?

If they have difficulty in any of these areas, refer them to an OT for a full assessment and treatment plan. Remember when obtaining this information that collateral information from the family is vital in order to obtain a clear picture of what the patient does during the day.

It may be necessary to educate the family on the patient's inability to perform at the standard at which they performed before they became ill. It is important that the family understands that this is not because the person is lazy or difficult, but because they are now unable to organize themselves as well as they used to. They may need assistance with organizing their day before they are able to manage themselves.

If you have any questions regarding a person's functioning, the best course to follow is to contact the local OT in your clinic or at the nearest hospital.

25 Psychopharmacology and nursing

At this stage according to law, registered nurses are not allowed to prescribe any of the psychotropic medications in South Africa. However, this may change in the future and it is crucial that nurses know the effects, side-effects, and management of side-effects in order to facilitate effective nursing interventions for patients and their families. This will also enhance patient compliance.

EDL (essential drugs list) for psychiatry in South Africa

Table 25.1 lists the drugs on the Essential Drugs List for use in psychiatry.

Table 25.1 Essential drugs list

- Chlorpromazine tablets, 25 mg, 100 mg (Largactil)
- Haloperidol IV/IM 5 mg/ml and tablets 5 mg (Serenace)
- Fluphenazine decanoate IM 25 mg/ml (Modecate)
- Flupenthixol depot IM 20 mg/ml (Fluanxol)

- Clothiapine injection 40 mg/4 mℓ (Etomine)
- Zuclopenthixol Acetate IM 50 mg/mℓ (Clopixol Acuphase) must be refrigerated
- Lorazepam IV/IM 4 mg/mℓ (Ativan) must be refrigerated
- Oxazepam tablets 10 mg, 15 mg (Serepax)
- Diazepam tablets 2 mg, 5 mg, 10 mg (Valium)
- Amitriptyline tablets 25 mg (Tryptanol)
- Imipramine tablets 10 mg, 25 mg (Tofranil)
- Fluoxetine capsules 20 mg (Prozac)
- Orphenadrine hydrochloride tablets 50 mg (Disipal)
- Biperiden injection 5 mg/mℓ (Akineton)

For delirium and status epilepticus:
- Diazepam injection 5 mg/mℓ (Valium)

As anti-epileptics/convulsants:
- Carbemazepine tablets 200 mg; syrup 100 mg/5 mℓ (Tegretol)
- Valproate tablets 200 mg, 500 mg, liquid 200 mg/5 mℓ (Epilim)

These drugs should be available in all PHC clinics. They are all Schedule 5 drugs and can only be prescribed by a doctor. However, nurses can still do the follow-up visit, and refer the patient to the doctor for medication. Even if these drugs are not currently available in PHC clinics, patients attending community mental health clinics may also attend the PHC clinics with physical complaints, and primary health care workers need to know the effects, side-effects, and interactions of these psychotropic drugs, as well as how to manage their side-effects.

Choice of treatment

The choice of a treatment should take account of the patient's past history, current clinical condition, and the treatment goals. Before starting a treatment, the clinician should have an idea of:

- the expected result;
- the time involved;
- strategies to deal with the side-effects expected;
- contingency plans should the chosen treatment fail; and
- whether long-term maintenance is indicated.

The patient's prior treatment history is a key guide in treatment selection. Factors to consider include response, side-effects, and compliance. A family history of response to an agent for a similar condition is a useful guide.

Monotherapy should always be the goal of a therapeutic regimen. Multiple drugs are associated with interactions and can cause confusion as to which of a series of agents is responsible for either a clinical effect or side-effects.

No treatment will work if patient compliance is inadequate. Factors that determine compliance include:

- the relationship with the prescriber;
- education regarding the illness;
- expected side-effects;
- duration of treatment; and
- the complexity of the treatment regime.

The greater the dose frequency and the larger the number of drugs, the worse compliance will be.

Medical conditions may be the cause of the presenting psychiatric illness. Drug interactions with medical therapy may either increase toxicity or decrease the effectiveness of prescribed psychotropics. Drug or alcohol abuse is likely to confound both diagnosis and treatment, and needs to be excluded. The elderly frequently need lower doses than younger adults. Dose changes in the elderly should be less frequent because these patients need more time to reach a steady state.

It is important to discontinue treatments that prove ineffective. A common mistake is to add new drugs to a failed regimen. This increases cost and potential toxicity without a corresponding increase in efficacy. When a drug is discontinued, it is prudent to taper the dose gradually. This reduces the risk of withdrawal effects. Withdrawal effects need to be distinguished from recurrence or relapse of a disorder following discontinuation of a maintenance treatment.

Polypharmacy should be minimized or excluded. Elderly patients and patients with illnesses that reduce drug protein binding, metabolism, and excretion generally need one-third to one-half of the usual therapeutic dosage of antidepressants. The use of fixed combination drugs is to be strongly discouraged.

Antidepressants

Table 25.2 Classification of antidepressants

I Tricyclic antidepressants
Trimipramine (Surmontil)
Amitriptyline (Tryptanol)*
Imipramine (Tofranil)*
Dothiepin (Prothiaden)
Clomipramine (Anafranil)
Maprotiline (Ludiomil)
Nortriptyline (Aventyl)
Desipramine (Pertofran)
Lofepramine (Emdalen)

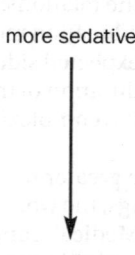

more sedative

less sedative

II Selective serotonin re-uptake inhibitors (SSRIs)
Fluoxetine (Prozac)*
Paroxetine (Aropax)
Citalopram (Cipramil)
Fluvoxamine (Luvox)
Sertraline (Zoloft)

III Other
Mianserin (Lantanon)
Traxodone (Molipaxin)
Venlafaxine (Effexor)
Nefazodone (Serzone)

Table 25.2 continued

IV Monoamine oxidase inhibitors
Tranylcypromine (Parnate)

V Reversible inhibitors of MAOA (RIMA)
Moclobemide (Aurorix)

*EDL

Pharmacological treatment and electroconvulsive therapy (ECT) have greatly improved the management of people afflicted with any of the major mood disorders. Pharmacotherapy does not replace a proper physical evaluation and history of the illness, nor does it exclude social manipulation, supportive therapy, or eventually psychotherapy.

Many compounds with diverse mechanisms of actions have antidepressant properties. In addition, many conditions as diverse as bulimia, tension headache, enuresis, and obsessive-compulsive disorder are relieved by antidepressants.

To date there is no single antidepressant excelling the others in antidepressant efficacy. The major differences between the agents are in the area of side-effects and toxicity.

Mechanisms of action

The immediate effect of most antidepressants is to increase the synaptic availability of monoamine neurotransmitters. The symptoms of depression begin to decrease after ten to twenty-one days of antidepressant treatment, at which time a number of alterations in receptor sensitivity occur. These include down-regulation of adrenergic beta 1 and alpha 2 receptors, and of serotonin 2 receptors, although changes in a large number of receptor systems, including acetylcholine, dopamine, and GABA, have been documented.

Indications for antidepressants

Antidepressants are useful in a variety of conditions, including the various forms of depression, many anxiety disorders, and other syndromes that are symptomatically far removed from depression.

Both acute treatment and relapse prevention of depression are the primary indications for the antidepressants, and 70 to 80 per cent of depressed patients respond to treatment as opposed to 30 to 40 per cent of patients who are given placebos.

The most common reasons for drug failure are inadequate dosage (less than 150 mg of a tricyclic, for example imipramine or equivalent) and length of treatment (six weeks).

Antidepressants are useful in the depressive phase of bipolar disorder, although they may induce both mania and rapid mood cycling in patients with bipolar disorder. Atypical depression, characterized by hyperphagia, hypersomnia, reverse diurnal mood variation (worse in the evenings), and rejection hypersensitivity, may respond preferentially to the monoamine oxidase (MAO) inhibitors.

Patients with psychotic depression typically need a combination of an antidepressant and an antipsychotic or ECT. Anxiety (including panic attacks) is a core feature of depression and anxious, depressed patients usually respond favourably to standard antidepressant therapy. Imipramine, MAOIs and SSRIs are all of documented efficacy in the treatment of panic disorder. The stimulating effects of the antidepressants in panic disorder are managed by starting at low doses and gradually increasing the dosage. Dysthymia, depression secondary to medical conditions, and depression co-morbid with substance abuse are also indications for antidepressant treatment.

The concept of reactive depression is of little value, as the fact that the depression is 'understandable' does little to help the sufferer. The decision to use an antidepressant should be based on symptom severity, with the presence of vegetative features suggesting the need for somatic therapy. Social and psychological factors should be addressed in all depressed patients.

Obsessive-compulsive disorder is responsive to serotonergic antidepressants, including clomipramine and the SSRIs. Higher doses in the order of 40–80 mg per day of fluoxetine

(Prozac) or 150–300 mg daily of clomipramine (Anafranil) are indicated, and trials in the order of three months are usually necessary.

Other conditions that are potentially responsive to antidepressants include post-traumatic stress disorder, social phobia (MAO inhibitors especially RIMAs, and fluoxetine), Bulimia (fluoxetine, tricyclics, MAO inhibitors), attention-deficit disorder (imipramine), chronic pain including tension headache (amitriptyline, imipramine, SSRIs), and enuresis (imipramine).

Choice of antidepressant

Factors influencing antidepressant choice include:
- previous response;
- family history of response;
- agitation (use sedative agent);
- motor retardation (use stimulating agent);
- cost;
- obsessive features (use serotonergic agent); and
- atypical depression (use MAOI).

In patients with a history of cardiac disease, the tricyclic agents (with the exception of lofepramine) should be avoided as they cause conduction changes and postural hypotension. In patients with epilepsy, tricyclics, particularly maprotiline and clomipramine, should be avoided. In patients with glaucoma or prostatism, the anticholinergic agents (tricyclics) should be avoided. The tricyclic agents (except lofepramine) are toxic in overdose, and should not be given to out-patients if suicidal ideation is present.

The minimum antidepressant course is six months after a single depressive episode, although patients who have had multiple episodes of depression will need longer periods of prophylactic antidepressant treatment. On discontinuation, antidepressants should be tapered rather than stopped abruptly.

Tricyclic antidepressants

Use

Because of their sedative properties and long half-life (forty-eight to seventy-two hours) tricyclics should be given as a single night-time dose. Due to their side-effects, it is best to start at lower doses (25–50 mg at night) and increase by 25 mg approximately every three days to about 150 mg daily. The dose should be titrated upward in accordance with side-effects and clinical response.

All antidepressants have a lag phase of at least two weeks before any significant antidepressant effects emerge, with full therapeutic response taking six to eight weeks or even longer. An adequate trial is therefore at least six weeks, after which a patient who shows no response should be given another agent, usually from another class.

Side-effects

The most serious problem is the issue of lethality in overdose. Doses of over 1 gram are potentially lethal, with death from uncontrolled seizures, arrhythmias, or hypotension.

Anticholinergic side-effects are common problems. A central anticholinergic syndrome is common in elderly, debilitated patients and those who are already on anticholinergic medication. Symptoms include agitation, confusion, memory impairment, hallucinations, and delirium. It is important to recognize these symptoms, as they may overlap with those of the primary condition and thus go unrecognized. Autonomic nervous system anticholinergic effects are common and include:

- blurred vision;
- dry mouth;
- urinary hesitancy and retention occurring mainly in males;
- tachycardia;
- aggravation of glaucoma; and
- constipation.

Sedative side-effects are common. Night-time dosing is essential and patients must be warned about driving, working with dangerous machinery, and the cumulative effect of sedative or hypnotic drugs and alcohol.

All the tricyclic antidepressants are epileptogenic. The most epileptogenic are maprotiline and clomipramine. There is no sound evidence regarding either clear risks or safety of the tricyclics in pregnancy. They are excreted into breast milk, although the implications of this are unclear.

Sexual side-effects include decreased libido, delayed or occasionally absent ejaculation or impotence in males, and orgasmic dysfunction in females. Increased sweating is common. Increased appetite, mainly in the form of carbohydrate craving with weight gain may occur.

Cardiovascular side-effects include hypotension and orthostatic hypotension, which are mediated by alpha 1 receptor blockade. Sinus tachycardias, supraventricular tachycardias, prolongation of the PR, QRS, and QT intervals, bundle branch and first-, second-, and third-degree heart blocks, as well as ST and T wave changes are documented (quinidine-like effects). These properties make their use in patients with myocardial damage or conduction defects dangerous, and patients receiving anaesthesia are at some risk. Contra-indications to the use of tricyclic antidepressants include recent myocardial infarct, atrio-ventricular conduction, disurbances or other significant cardiac disease.

The selective serotonin re-uptake inhibitors (SSRIs)

Use

The SSRIs have rapidly become one of the first-line agents in the treatment of depression. This is due to the absence of anticholinergic and cardiac side-effects, safety in overdose, and absence of weight gain in their use. The SSRIs include fluoxetine, citalopram, sertraline, paroxetine, and fluvoxamine. The oldest SSRI, namely fluoxetine, is well established for the treatment of depression, OCD, bulimia and panic disorder, as well as generalized anxiety disorder and premenstrual syndrome.

As most of the SSRIs except fluvoxamine are non-sedative, they are best used as a single morning dose; fluvoxamine should be given in the evening. The standard dose for the treatment of depression is 20 mg daily for fluoxetine, citalopram, and paroxetine, 50 mg daily for sertraline, and 100 mg daily for fluvoxamine. Given their tolerability, the SSRIs can usually be started at the necessary dose. In panic disorder, however, it is prudent to start at lower doses, and gradually increase the dose, as the stimulatory properties of the SSRIs may initially agitate some patients. Bulimia and OCD may require higher doses in the 60–80 mg daily range of fluoxetine or its equivalent.

Side-effects

The most common side-effects of the SSRIs include nausea, restlessness, insomnia, headaches, and diarrhoea. Insomnia may respond to low (50–100 mg) doses of trazodone. most of these side-effects tend to be transient. Sexual dysfunction, including anorgasmia, ejaculatory delay, and reduced libido, is common.

Monoamine oxidase inhibitors (MAOIs)

The only MAOI currently available is tranylcypromine. Due to the irreversible inhibition of both the A and B forms of MAO, ingested catecholamines such as tyramine enter the bloodstream and can cause a potentially fatal hypertensive reaction – the so-called cheese reaction. The symptoms of this hyperadrenergic crisis include severe hypertension, hyperpyrexia, and other signs of sympathetic overactivity.

Patients on the old MAOIs must be on a tyramine-free diet from ten days prior to taking the first tablet and stay on the diet until fourteen days after the last tablet to prevent a possible hypertensive crisis. A hypertensive crisis may also occur with vasoconstrictors. A variety of medication may have potentially fatal interactions with MAOIs, for example pethidine and the SSRIs.

Because of their potentially serious side-effects, these are definitely not the first line of antidepressant treatment. They are usually reserved for patients who fail to respond to conventional antidepressants. The MAOIs may also be particularly useful in patients with atypical depression or panic.

Compliant patients, however, may benefit greatly from this drug.

Tranylcypromine (Parnate) should be started slowly, building up by 10 mg once or twice a week to reach a dose of approximately 30 mg twice a day, although doses of up to 80 mg a day are sometimes necessary. Side-effects include the cheese effect, postural hypotension, insomnia, agitation, and sexual dysfunction.

Psychoeducation for antidepressants

Table 25.3 Tricyclic antidepressants: educational plan

Provide the patient with the following information:
Dry mouth
- Rinse mouth with water.
- Brush teeth more frequently.
- Chew sugarless sweets or gum.
- Apply lip balm to lips and nostrils.

Nausea, vomiting, poor appetite
- Eat crackers, toast, drink tea.
- Drink protein supplement to maintain weight.

Weight gain
- Eat less sugar, starch, and fat.
- Increase protein intake.
- Exercise daily.
- Follow a diet prescribed by doctor.

Personal-hygiene and body temperature
Decrease of normal bacteria in mouth may result in infection
- Avoid foods high in sugar.
- Observe tongue for signs of thick white coating.
- Increase mouth care, including brushing tongue and gargling with mouthwash.

Table 25.3 continued

Increased sensitivity to the heat and decreased sweating
- Shower in lukewarm water.
- Avoid exertion in hot weather.
- Dress appropriately for environmental conditions.
- Take own oral temperature.
- Avoid temperature extremes such as hot tubs.

Greater chance of a bad sunburn
- Use sunscreen and lip balm when out in the sun.
- Wear clothes that protect skin, including a hat.
- Wear sunglasses.

Vaginal dryness
- Use a lubricant such as K-Y jelly.

Menstrual period may stop
- Notify nurse and doctor.
- Continue to use birth control.

General changes in interest in sex
- Notify nurse and doctor.

Decreased moisture around eyes
- Use extra caution if contact lenses are worn, in order to avoid eye irritation.

Dizziness
- Lie down and rest.
- Get up slowly from lying position, dangle legs over edge of bed.
- Have nurse check blood pressure.

Difficulty urinating
- Drink 6 to 8 glasses of fluid each day.
- Notify nurse and doctor.
- Do relaxation exercises to promote urination.
- Apply warm water to genital area.

Table 25.3 continued

- Take a lukewarm shower.
- Listen to running water.

Constipation
- Drink 6 to 8 glasses of fluid each day.
- Eat green vegetables and bran each day.
- Exercise daily.
- Eat prunes or raisins.
- Take laxative medication only with a doctor's advice.
- Notify nurse and doctor.

Drowsiness
- Drive car or other vehicles with extra care.
- Avoid alcoholic beverages or street drugs.
- Plan for extra rest time.
- Avoid other medications unless approved by a doctor.

Muscle tightness/cramping in arms, legs, neck, or face
- Notify nurse and doctor.
- Take medications for side-effects.

Compulsion to keep moving and inability to sit down; restlessness
- Notify nurse and doctor.
- Take medication for side-effects.

Blurred vision
- Use a magnifying glass for reading.

Eye pain in sunlight
- Wear sunglasses when outside.

Understanding of illness and medication
- Talk with nurse and doctor to identify symptoms that are part of the illness or side-effects from the medication.

Decreased interest in surroundings and usual activities
- Discuss this feeling with nurse or doctor.

A psychoeducation plan for all antidepressants will be very similar and this plan can be adapted for use.

Mood stabilizers

The following drugs are used in the treatment of bipolar disorder (manic-depressive illness) to prevent relapses of either mania or depression (as this is a chronic illness, the person needs life-long treatment):

- lithium carbonate (note: not on the EDL);
- carbamazepine*;
- valproic acid*;

(*on the EDL)

Lithium carbonate

The usual dose is 400–800 mg daily, but this depends on how well the person's kidneys are functioning. Anyone on this drug needs to have their blood checked at least every three months, as this drug is extremely dangerous in overdose. Therefore it should only be prescribed where there are adequate laboratory facilities to check lithium levels. There are certain conditions that can increase the amount of lithium in the body to dangerous levels:

- any case of dehydration (gastro-enteritis, heavy exercise in hot conditions);
- use of diuretics; or
- renal problems (infection, renal failure).

Use

- Acute manic states. Lithium controls motor hyperactivity, elation, talkativeness, flight of ideas, and restlessness.
- Prophylactic use in recurrent manic-depressive episodes.

Absorption: Lithium is rapidly absorbed after oral administration, reaching peak serum levels in one to four hours. Transient nausea, fine hand tremor, diarrhoea, thirst, and polyuria may be associated with serum lithium peaks.

These symptoms appear to be related to the steepness

of dosage, and diminish without reduction of dosage. Therapeutic effect does not occur until seven to ten days after initiating dosage. In the treatment of acute manic states the patient may be given a combination of an antipsychotic drug such as chlorpromazine (Largactil) and lithium.

Excretion: Lithium is excreted almost exclusively through the kidneys. There is a relationship between sodium intake and lithium excretion. Lithium is excreted more rapidly when there is a high sodium intake and less rapidly when there is a low sodium intake. When sodium depletion occurs, it can promote lithium retention, which enhances lithium toxicity and may produce rapid development of side-effects. It is for this reason that lithium should be administered only to patients with normal sodium intake.

Renal lithium clearance decreases with advancing age; therefore elderly patients require smaller doses of lithium to maintain the same serum lithium level as younger adults.

Action

- Antimanic without producing sedation.
- Lithium alters sodium transport in nerve and muscle cells; however, specific mechanism of lithium action in manic states is unknown.

Side-effects

Minor lithium toxicity: These side-effects usually subside during the first few weeks of treatment with lithium. When symptoms persist, temporary reduction of dosage or discontinuance of lithium will result in cessation of symptoms. Symptoms include:

- fine hand tremor;
- transient nausea;
- fatigue;
- thirst;
- polyuria;
- diarrhoea; and
- muscle weakness.

Major lithium toxicity: The onset of lithium toxicity is usually gradual, and is an indication for discontinuing the drug. Note:

- coarse tremor;
- sluggishness;
- lassitude;
- drowsiness;
- confusion;
- slurred speech;
- ataxia;
- vomiting;
- diarrhoea;
- impaired consciousness; and
- coma.

Psychoeducation for lithium carbonate

Table 25.4 Nursing interventions for lithium carbonate

Initial symptoms of nausea
- Take lithium with meals or with food in the stomach:
- Drink tea or broth and eat soda crackers.

Worsening of symptoms of nausea or vomiting
- Notify nurse and physician.
- Do not take the next dose of lithium before consulting with the nurse and/or physician.
- Do not diet unless specifically prescribed by a physician.

Increased urination
- Drink 6 to 8 glasses of fluid each day.
- Notify nurse and/or physician.

Diarrhoea
- Maintain fluid intake.
- Notify nurse and/or physician.

Skin breakdown due to swelling
- Elevate legs when swelling is present.
- Maintain good personal hygiene.

Table 25.4 continued

Sweating my affect the lithium level
- Avoid exposure to changes in temperature.
- Wear clothes appropriate to the temperature.
- Maintain fluid and salt intake.

Increased sweating due to exercise
- Wear clothes appropriate to the temperature.
- Maintain fluid and salt intake.
- Do not change exercise habits without discussion with nurse and physician.

Difficulty urinating
- Drink 6 to 8 glasses of fluid each day.
- Notify nurse and doctor.
- Do relaxation exercises to promote urination.
- Apply warm water to genital area.
- Take a lukewarm shower.
- Listen to running water.

Constipation
- Drink 6 to 8 glasses of fluid each day.
- Eat green vegetables and bran each day.
- Exercise daily.
- Eat prunes or raisins.
- Take laxative medication only with doctor's advice.
- Notify nurse and doctor.

Drowsiness
- Drive cars or other vehicles with extra care.
- Avoid alcoholic beverages or street drugs.
- Plan for extra rest time.
- Avoid other medications unless approved by a doctor.

Muscle tightness/cramping in arms, legs, neck, or face
- Notify nurse and doctor.
- Take medications for side-effects.

Table 25.4 continued

Compulsion to keep moving and inability to sit down; restlessness
- Notify nurse and doctor.
- Take medication for side-effects.

Blurred vision
- Use a magnifying glass for reading.

Eye pain in sunlight
- Wear sunglasses when outside.

Understanding of illness and medication
- Talk with nurse and doctor to identify symptoms that are part of the illness or side-effects from medication.

Decreased interest in surroundings and usual activities
- Discuss this feeling with the doctor.

Carbamazepine and valproic acid

These are second line treatments where lithium has either failed or is contra-indicated. As these are coded as anticonvulsants they are on the EDL and will be available at PHC clinics.

Carbamazepine

Carbamazepine has been shown to be of use both in the treatment of mania and in prophylaxis of bipolar disorder, particularly rapid cycling and affective symptoms secondary to seizure disorders. The usual dose of carbamazepine is 600–1000 mg daily and build up to a therapeutic dose, increasing by 100 mg every day or two to minimize side-effects.

Serious side-effects such as hepatitis, exfoliative dermatitis (Stevens-Johnson Syndrome), and blood dyscrasias are extremely rare. The most common side-effects are neurological and include sedation, vertigo, blurred vision, and ataxia. Although insignificant decreases in white cell counts are frequent, agranulocytosis and aplastic anaemia are extremely rare. Nausea and vomiting, slowing of cardiac conduction, rash (urticaria and pruritic erythematous rashes), and hyponatraemia are other documented side-effects.

Valproic acid

Valproic acid is used in the treatment of mania, with some evidence of utility in prophylaxis of bipolar disorder. The dose should be commenced slowly at 200 mg daily and increased every few days to about 1600–1800 mg in three divided doses. Sedation, nausea, and vomiting are common problems, and other side-effects include raised liver enzymes, tremor, and platelet dysfunction.

Psychoeducation for carbamazepine

Table 25.5 Psychoeducation for carbamazepine

Dry mouth
- Rinse mouth with water.
- Brush teeth more frequently.
- Chew sugarless sweets/gum.
- Apply lip balm to lips and nostrils.
- Drink 6 to 8 glasses of fluid each day.

Difficulty urinating
- Apply warm water to genital area.
- Take a lukewarm shower.
- Listen to running water.

Diarrhoea
- Maintain fluid intake.
- Notify nurse and/or physician.

Possible inflammation of the tongue and lining of the mouth
- Notify physician or nurse immediately.

Table 25.5 continued

- Use a soft bristle toothbrush.
- Rinse mouth frequently.
- Avoid foods that contain spices such as pepper, nutmeg, or vinegar.

Possible rash/itching skin
- Notify nurse or doctor.
- Apply lotions to skin.
- Do no use soaps that dry the skin.

Nausea/vomiting, poor appetite
- Notify nurse and physician.
- Eat soda crackers, toast; drink tea.

Dizziness
- Lie down and rest.
- Get up slowly from a lying position; dangle legs over edge of bed for 5 minutes before standing up.
- Have nurse check blood pressure.

Drowsiness
- Drive car or other vehicles with extra care.
- Avoid alcoholic beverages or street drugs.
- Plan for extra rest time.

Blurred vision
- Notify nurse or physician.
- Use a magnifying glass for reading.

Understanding the illness and medications
- Talk with nurse and physician to identify symptoms that are part of the illness or side-effects from medication.

Benzodiazepines and other anxiolytics and hypnotics

Table 25.6 Classification of benzodiazepines according to eliminaton half-life of the parent compound and active metabolites

Ultra-short half-life (less than 6 hours)
Midazolam (Dormicum)
Triazolam (Halcion)

Short half-life (6 to 12 hours)
Zopiclone (Imovane)
Lormetazepam (Noctamid)
Loprazolam (Dormonoct)
Oxazepam (Serepax)*
Temazepam (Normison)

Intermediate half-life (12 to 24 hours)
Alprazolam (Xanor)
Bromazepam (Lexotan)
Lorazepam (Ativan)
Quazepam (Dorme)

Long half-life (more than 24 hours)
Chlordiazepoxide (Librium)
Clobazam (Urbanol)
Clonazepam (Rivotril)
Clorazepate (Traxene)
Diazepam (Valium)*
Flunitrazepam (Rohypnol)
Flurazepam (Dalmadorm)
Nitrazepam (Mogadon)
Prazepam (Demetrin)
*EDL

Use

Over the past thirty years benzodiazepines with their low LD50 and wide therapeutic margin have replaced the barbiturates and are extensively prescribed. There has been some decline in the prescription of benzodiazepines in the last few years. This is due to decreased symptomatic prescription in conditions such as depression and the introduction of new classes of non-benzodiazepine compounds. These include both anxiolytics like the azapirones such as buspirone and cyclopyrrolone hypnotics including zopiclone.

Indications

All the benzodiazepines have sedative/hypnotic, muscle relaxant, anxiolytic, anticonvulsant, and amnestic properties. Indications include anxiety disorders, including generalized anxiety disorders, adjustment disorders with anxious mood and anticipatory anxiety, and also anxiety secondary to another psychiatric and physical illness. Sleep disorders, particularly primary and secondary insomnia disorders, respond to judicious use of hypnotics as do withdrawal states, especially from alcohol. PRN ('as needed') prescription in psychotic agitation, depression, and panic disorder is useful.

Side-effects

- drowsiness;
- fatigue;
- dizziness;
- ataxia;
- blurred vision;
- slurred speech;
- tremor; and
- hypotension.

The benzodiazepines may induce tolerance, dependence, and the risk of withdrawal reactions on discontinuation. Pharmacokinetic factors in dependence risk include:
- long-term treatment;
- higher dosage;

- high-potency drugs (e.g. midazolam, flunitrazepam, alprazolam, lorazepam); and
- drugs with a short duration of action (e.g. midazolam, triazolam, alprazolam).

Short half-life drugs with low potency (e.g. zopiclone, oxazepam, and temazepam) and long half-life drugs with low potency (e.g. chlordiazepoxide and diazepam) are associated with a lower dependence risk. Delirium, seizures, and dysphoria can occur, particularly after discontinuation of the short-acting high-potency agents. It is often useful to convert patients from these agents onto a low-potency, long-acting drug in order to facilitate drug withdrawal.

In the elderly, accumulation, particularly of the longer-acting drugs, is associated with an increased risk of hip fractures. Low-potency short-acting agents such as oxazepam and temazepam are safest. Due to equivocal evidence of facial cleft defects and intrauterine growth restriction, use in pregnancy needs to be avoided unless compelling indications are present.

Fatigue, drowsiness, and impaired psychomotor co-ordination are common side-effects. These are dose dependent, and dissipate with the development of tolerance. Particularly the short-acting high-potency agents such as midazolam and triazolam are associated with impairment of recent memory. Disinhibition of behaviour with the benzodiazepines is described. Aggravation of depression is another described side-effect. Benzodiazepines are remarkably safe in overdose.

Psychoeducation for benzodiazepines

Table 25.7 Psychoeducation for benzodiazepines

Food in the stomach will slow the absorption of this medicine

- Do not take medication with meals.
- If stomach upset is present, drink tea and broth and take soda crackers.
- Notify nurse or physician if other stomach problems arise.

Table 25.7 continued

Effectiveness of this drug is lessened with excessive intake of caffeine or heavy tobacco smoking.

- Drink decaffeinated beverages; avoid caffeinated colas, chocolate, or tea.
- Keep smoking to a minimum, if possible.

Alcohol increases the sedating effects of this drug

- Alcohol intake is not permitted during hospitalization.
- Avoid alcohol after discharge, if continuing with the medication.

Possible rash/itching skin

- Notify nurse or physician.
- Apply lotions to skin.
- Do not use soap that dries skin.

Dizziness

- Lie down and rest.
- Get up slowly from lying position, dangle legs over edge of bed.
- Have nurse check blood pressure.
- Notify physician or nurse.

Difficulty urinating

- Drink 6 to 8 glasses of fluid each day.
- Notify nurse and physician.
- Do relaxation exercises to promote urination.
- Apply warm water to genital area.
- Take a lukewarm shower.
- Listen to running water.

Constipation

- Drink 6 to 8 glasses of fluid each day.
- Eat green vegetables and bran each day.
- Exercise daily.
- Eat prunes or raisins.
- Take laxative medication only with a doctor's advice.

Table 25.7 continued

Drowsiness
- Drive cars or other vehicles with extra care.
- Plan for extra rest time.
- Avoid other medications unless approved by a physician.

Blurred vision
- Notify nurse or doctor.
- Use a magnifying glass for reading.

Unusual irritability or nervousness
- Notify physician or nurse.
- Ask nurse for assistance in selecting an appropriate relaxation exercise.

Understanding the illness and medications
- Talk with nurse and physician to identify symptoms that are part of the illness or side-effects from the medication.

Hypnotics

Use
- insomnia;
- anxiety and tension states;
- preoperative sedation;
- alcohol withdrawal; and
- control of convulsive seizures.

There are many reasons why people have trouble sleeping. Often there is some stress in the person's life. Once this is resolved the person sleeps normally again. Some people sleep poorly all the time. This may be due to some physical illness or due to chronic stress or a psychiatric illness.

Certain simple measures can also help a person to sleep at night, e.g. a hot drink (not alcohol – this disrupts sleep), a routine bedtime if possible, some relaxing activity before going to sleep, a light snack. If this does not help and the person's daytime functioning is being affected by poor sleep, then a sedative could be prescribed. However, this should only be given for a short period, for example three weeks, and if possible, every two to three nights. This is to avoid the problem of addiction, as sedatives are highly addictive.

Diazepam 5 mg at night, or oxazepam 10–20 mg at night.

Actions

- produces sedation;
- produces sleep;
- produces anticonvulsive activity; and
- produces respiratory depression.

Side-effects

- drowsiness;
- dizziness;
- ataxia;
- impaired judgment;
- slurred speech;
- headache;
- nausea and vomiting;
- diarrhoea;
- drug hangover (depression, lassitude, headache); and
- skin rash.

Paradoxial reactions of excitement and confusion are rare, and most likely to occur in the elderly.

Psychoeducation for hypnotics

Table 25.8 Nursing interventions for hypnotics

- Advise patients not to drink alcohol when taking sedatives and hypnotics. Additive CNS depression occurs when alcohol is taken with sedative and hypnotic drugs.

Table 25.8 continued

- Hypnotics and sedatives should never be left at the bedside. Stay with the patient until the drug has been taken.
- To avoid accidental ingestion by the patient or children, advise patients not to keep hypnotics and sedatives in a bedside table.
- Sedatives and hypnotics are not analgesics. Restlessness and excitement may result if administered to patients in severe pain.
- Narcotic analgesics and sedative-hypnotics are CNS depressants and should not be administered together, unless the physician is consulted. Adjustment of dosage may be required.
- Institute nursing measures to promote comfort and sleep before administering a hypnotic. Some patients are not able to sleep because of physical discomfort or anxiety and tension. Establishing a relaxing bedtime regimen may help to induce sleep.
- Observe sleep patterns. Type of sleep disturbance is a factor in determining which hypnotic drug will be effective.
- Elderly patients may become restless, confused, and disoriented. Observe the response to the drug and institute safety precautions such as side rails and assistance with ambulation, if necessary.
- Advise patients not to drive or operate dangerous machinery, since impairment of judgment and fine motor skills may persist for many hours following administration of sedatives and hypnotics.
- Check with the physician before administering a sedative if the patient appears excessively drowsy.
- Advise patients to take sedatives and hypnotics exactly as pre-scribed. The dose should never be increased without consulting the physician. These drugs should not be discontinued abruptly as with-drawal symptoms such as muscular weakness, anxiety, insomnia, tremors, and convulsions may occur.
- Barbiturates depress the respiratory centre and have been used for suicide. Barbiturate supply should be limited and carefully safe-guarded.

Antipsychotic agents

Table 25.9 Antipsychotic equivalent doses

Low-potency agents

Chlorpromazine (Largactil) 200–400 mg daily

Clozapine (Leponex) 200–400 mg daily

Sulpiride (Eglonyl) 400–800 mg daily

High-potency agents

Haloperidol (Serenace) 5–10 mg daily*

Trifluoperazine (Stelazine) 5–20 mg daily

Pimozide (Orap) 2–4 mg daily

Risperidone (Risperdal) 4–6 mg daily

Olanzapine (Zyprexa) 10 mg daily

Quetiapine (Seroquel) dose titrated to 300–450 mg daily

Depot preparations

Flupenthixol (Fluanxol) 40 mg two- to three-weekly*

Zuclopenthixol (Clopixol) 100 mg four-weekly*

Fluphenazine (Modecate) 25 mg four-weekly*

*EDL

Use

Antipsychotics are usefully divided into high- and low-potency agents. It is important to understand that the efficacy of these drugs is the same; potency refers to the dose required. In principle, the low-potency agents tend to be more sedating, and have more anticholinergic and non-adrenergic alpha-blocking properties, while the high-potency agents have more neurological side-effects. All antipsychotics are dopamine antagonists, with most antipsychotics acting as blockers of the D2 receptor, although certain agents have antagonistic properties at D1 and D4 receptors as well. Although the blockade is immediate, antipsychotic response usually takes at least ten days.

The antipsychotics tend to be available in oral and in both short- and long-acting (depot) parenteral forms. Due to first pass metabolism, a much lower parenteral than oral dose needs to be administered.

Indications

Antipsychotic drugs have a wide range of efficacy in a substantial number of psychotic conditions, particularly schizophrenia. However, there is evidence that the antipsychotics are more useful for the positive than for the negative symptoms of this illness, although claims are made for the efficacy of the atypical antipsychotics clozapine, risperidone, olanzapine, and quetiapine in the treatment of negative symptoms. Antipsychotics are used not only for acute exacerbation of schizophrenia, but also for the long-term maintenance or prophylactic treatment of schizophrenic patients.

Although lithium alone is sufficient for a mild manic episode, the antipsychotics are the agents of choice for more severe manic behaviour, particularly if psychotic symptoms are present. Patients suffering from psychotic depressive episodes require an antipsychotic in combination with an antidepressant. An alternative treatment is ECT. The antipsychotics are useful in the treatment of schizo-affective disorder, schizophreniform disorder, and the delusional disorders. Low doses of the high-potency antipsychotics are occasionally useful in the treatment of the behavioural disorder associated with delirium and dementia. They are also used for movement disorders including Tourette's disorder and Huntington's disease.

It is essential to do a thorough assessment of every patient prior to the initiation of antipsychotics. These agents should not be used for treatment of non-specific symptoms such as anxiety, which may be better treated by other agents. There are three major situations in which antipsychotics are used:

- acute psychosis in which the behaviour constitutes a medical emergency;
- long-term treatment of chronic psychotic disorders; and
- the use of antipsychotics on an 'as needed' (PRN) basis.

Haloperidol doses of 5–10 mg, chlorpromazine dosages of 200–400 mg a day, or equivalent are sufficient for the treatment of most psychotic illnesses. Higher doses tend to be associated with more side-effects, and lower doses with diminished efficacy. It is however, occasionally necessary to use higher doses in severely agitated, behaviourally disturbed patients, particularly manic patients. The addition of a high-potency benzodiazepine such as lorazepam under these circumstances is often useful in allowing sedation of highly agitated patients while allowing lower doses of antipsychotics to be used.

Because insight and motivation is often impaired in schizophrenia, depot preparations are frequently useful. The preparations currently available include fluphenazine, flupenthixol, and zuclopenthixol. The ease of use of these compounds makes them a first-line choice in the maintenance treatment of chronic schizophrenia. It is advisable that patients be initially given an oral preparation in order to assess the tolerability of these drugs.

Antipsychotics are commonly used for restraint. The agents commonly used for restraint include haloperidol 10–30 mg in divided doses, which can be administered by mouth, intramuscularly, or intravenously. If administered intravenously the injection should be slow and vital signs should be monitored (especially pulse rate and blood pressure). Clothiapine in divided doses of 20 mg to maximum 240 mg in twenty-four hours can be given similarly. Precautions and observation as for haloperidol should occur. Chlorpromazine should not be used as the drug of choice for restraint. However, it is so universally available that it may be the only agent at hand. Doses of 50 mg to 500 mg in divided doses can be given orally. (Chlorpromazine should not be given IV or IMI).

Most of the patients in this category are highly aroused, and should a patient be difficult to control, it is wise to add a benzodiazepine once the upper dose ranges of antipsychotic have been reached. It is safer to add a benzodiazepine than to administer very high doses of antipsychotic. Slow intravenous administration will mitigate against respiratory depression. The benzodiazepines commonly used are diazepam 5–40 mg, lorazepam 2–8 mg, or clonazepam 0,5–4 mg.

Choice of antipsychotic

Choice of agent is predominantly based on marrying the side-effect profile of the drug with the patient's clinical profile. It is useful to master the use of one or two high-and low-potency agents. A patient who has responded well to a particular agent in the past should be prescribed the same drug again. If a person has a history of extrapyramidal side-effects, the low-potency agents may be preferable. The low-potency agents are more dangerous in overdose, and suicidal patients should hence be given high-potency agents. Patients with glaucoma, prostatism, or other contraindications to anticholinergic drugs should not be given low-potency drugs, neither should these drugs be given to patients on other anticholinergic drugs such as tricyclic antidepressants.

Patients with a history of cardiac illness should be given high-potency agents and elderly patients should generally be given low doses of high-potency agents. Patients with Parkinson's disease should be given the low-potency agents or atypical antipsychotics. In the presence of delirium, the anticholinergic low-potency drugs should be avoided. In patients who have shown themselves to be refractory to conventional antipsychotics, clozapine and risperidone are possible alternatives.

Side-effects of antipsychotic medications

- neurological side-effects;
- sedation;
- hypertension;
- dry-mouth, blurred vision, urinary retention;
- skin reactions, including sensitivity of skin to sunlight;
- breast engorgement and inappropriate lactation;
- effects on blood cells; and
- jaundice.

Neurological side-effects

These drugs produce a syndrome that is called Parkinson's syndrome (Parkinsonism). It is similar to the disease known as Parkinson's disease. The symptoms and signs include the following:
- a feeling of stiffness, or of being slowed down;
- tremor;
- slow movements;
- expressionless face;
- slow, shuffling gait.
- increased muscle tone; and
- cog-wheel rigidity.

If a patient develops these side-effects, medication should be given as follows:
- biperiden (Akineton) 2–4 mg four times a day (*NB. Not on EDL*).
- orphenadrine (Disipal) 50–100 mg three times a day.

These are anticholinergic drugs, which reverse the Parkinsonian side-effects.

Acute dystonic reaction

The most likely side-effect to present as an emergency is an acute dystonic reaction. However, it usually presents within one to five days after starting on antipsychotic medication. It most commonly affects young male patients, and the drugs most likely to cause it are:
- haloperidol (Serenace);
- fluphenazine (Modecate);
- trifluoperazine (Stelazine); and
- flupenthixol (Fluanxol).

There is often a striking reaction, with spasm of the tongue, neck, and back muscles. There may be facial grimacing, and the eyes may deviate to one side. Patients may present with dysarthria (slurred or difficult speech) or dysphagia (difficulty in swallowing). They may dribble because they are unable to swallow even their own saliva. They may appear stiff, even catatonic. If they are unable to give a history, the presentation may be misinterpreted as being part of their psychiatric condition and more antipsychotics may be given. This will worsen the condition. *Immediate treatment with an anticholinergic agent such as biperiden (Akineton)* will alleviate the problem. If this is given intravenously, slowly, the recovery is dramatic. However, given intramuscularly, recovery usually occurs within half-an-hour. The dose given is usually 2,5–5 mg (0,5–1 mℓ). *Injectable biperiden is available on the Primary EDL.*

The patient must then be *referred* to hospital or to community psychiatry for further management, as her or his medication will probably need to be changed. The dose of the offending drug should be reduced and the patient should be given oral biperiden 2–4 mg six-hourly, or oral orphenadrine 50–100 mg six-hourly to prevent further problems.

Very rarely, there may be spasm of the laryngeal muscles too. Intravenous administration of biperiden may relieve the spasm. However, occasionally the spasm may persist even after this. If it is not possible to intubate the patient, an emergency tracheostomy must be performed to prevent asphyxiation. Basic resuscitation and life-support must be carried out, until the patient reaches hospital.

Akathisia

This is a side-effect that can be quite distressing to patients. They are very restless and cannot keep still. They may get up from sitting and pace, being unable to sit in a chair for any length of time. When they stand they often walk on the spot, and cannot keep their legs still.

It may be difficult to assess whether the person is restless because they are psychotic, or because of this side-effect of the medication. If you ask the person whether they feel the restlessness in their mind or in their body, they may be able to tell you which it is. If it is in their body, they are probably suffering from this side-effect. They need referral, as the medication may have to be reduced or changed.

Tardive dyskinesia (TD)

This is a serious long-term side-effect of antipsychotic medication. It is more likely to occur in the elderly, and in people who have been on antipsychotics for a long time. It consists of repetitive movements of the mouth, tongue, jaw, and neck. It can be distressing for the patient, and is certainly distressing for those around him or her. It may be *irreversible*. This emphasizes the need for using these medications only when indicated. Any patient on antipsychotics who develops this side-effect should be referred to community psychiatry for assessment as the medication may need to be changed or stopped. Sometimes one needs to continue medication despite the TD, if stopping the medication would be worse for the patient.

Psychoeducation for antipsychotic medication

Table 25.10 Nursing interventions for antipsychotic medication

Dry mouth
- Rinse mouth with water.
- Brush teeth more frequently.
- Chew sugarless sweets/gum.
- Apply lip balm to your lips and nostrils.

Nasal Stuffiness
- Avoid using OTC nasal sprays/drops.

Weight gain
- Eat less sugar, starch, and fat.
- Increase protein intake.
- Exercise daily.
- Follow a diet prescribed by a doctor.

Difficulty urinating
- Drink 6 to 8 glasses of fluid each day.
- Notify nurse and doctor.
- Do relaxation exercises to promote urination.
- Apply warm water to genital area.

Table 25.10 continued

- Take a lukewarm shower.
- Take own oral temperature.
- Avoid temperature extremes such as hot tubs.

Greater chance of a bad sunburn
- Use sunscreen and lip balm when out in the sun.
- Wear clothes that protect skin, including a hat.
- Wear sunglasses.

Vaginal dryness
- Use a lubricant such as K-Y jelly.

Menstrual period may stop
- Notify nurse and doctor.
- Continue to use birth control.

General changes in interest in sex
- Notify nurse and doctor.

Decreased moisture around eyes
- Use extra caution if contact lenses are worn, to avoid eye irritation.

Decrease of normal bacteria in mouth may result in infection
- Avoid foods high in sugar.
- Observe tongue for signs of thick white coating.
- Increase mouth care, including brushing tongue and gargling with mouthwash.

Increased sensitivity to the heat and decreased sweating
- Shower in lukewarm water.
- Avoid exertion in hot weather.
- Dress appropriately for environmental conditions.

Dizziness
- Lie down and rest.
- Get up slowly from lying position, dangle legs over edge of bed.
- Have nurse check blood pressure.

Table 25.10 continued

Constipation

- Drink 6 to 8 glasses of fluid each day.
- Eat green vegetables and bran each day.
- Exercise daily.
- Eat prunes or raisins.
- Take laxative medication only with a doctor's advice.
- Notify nurse and doctor.

Drowsiness

- Drive car or other vehicles with extra care.
- Avoid alcoholic beverages or street drugs.
- Plan for extra rest time.
- Avoid other medications unless approved by the physician.

Muscle tightness/cramping in arms, legs, neck, or face

- Notify nurse and doctor.
- Take medications for side-effects.

Compulsion to keep moving and inability to sit down; restlessness

- Notify nurse and doctor.
- Take medication for side-effects.

Blurred vision

- Use a magnifying glass for reading.

Eye pain in sunlight

- Wear sunglasses when outside.

Understanding of illness and medication

- Talk with nurse and doctor to identify symptoms that are part of the illness or side-effects from the medication.

Decreased interest in surroundings and usual activities

- Discuss this feeling with nurse or physician.

PART V
Legal framework within a PHC setting

26 Mental Health Act – implications for the primary mental health nurse

People who are mentally ill or challenged, or psychologically vulnerable in other respects may behave in a way that is detrimental to their health or lives, or they may become a danger to others. They frequently present without an appreciation of the need for help. There are specific laws to provide for the control and treatment of mentally ill people, for their own protection and for the protection of other members of the community.

Individuals suffering from psychiatric disorders may break laws because of:

- their lack of understanding;
- their disturbed perception of the world around them;
- their abnormal emotional state; or
- defects in intellect or personality.

The clinicians concerned are required to assist the legal system by offering appropriate recommendations for detainment or treatment in order to prevent repetition of the offence.

In order to do this, primary health care workers must have a basic understanding of the content and application of statutory laws affecting patients. The subspeciality in the area of interaction between psychiatry and the law is known as forensic psychiatry (medicolegal practice). The word 'forensic' is derived from *forum* (Latin), which means 'court' and implies that, in these cases, the interactions between the doctor and the patient are not private as is usually the case. The relevant law may be divided into civil and criminal aspects. The term 'forensic' generally refers to the criminal aspects.

All nurses in the primary health care setting function within the structures set out by the South African Nursing Council. When working with mentally ill persons, the nurse functions within the structure of the *Mental Health Act* 18 of 1973 (*MHA*), as amended. This act is currently being revised, and the new act should be in place before the end of 2001.

In the primary health care setting, mentally ill people occasionally require hospitalization when they do not realize that this is so. They become aggressive or violent as a result of their illness. In such circumstances, we say that they are a danger to others or to themselves. If they do not receive medical treatment for their illness, tragedies could occur, with loss of life or injury to themselves or others. Nurses should be aware of this and should understand the admission procedures and their implications.

Definitions

Medical workers and lawyers have different approaches to mental illness. Medical workers are concerned with the clinical setting and treatment procedures, while lawyers are responsible for following the due process of the law and its applications. Legal descriptions of various concepts may be different from descriptions used by doctors and nurses. The following common definitions are included in the *Mental Health Act* 18 of 1973 (*MHA*):

• Patient: 'A person mentally ill to such a degree that it is necessary that he be detained, supervised, controlled and

treated and includes a person who is suspected of being or is alleged to be mentally ill to such a degree'.
- Mental illness: 'Any disorder or disability of the mind, and includes any mental illness, any arrested or incomplete development of the mind'.

Hospitalization for treatment

(See Table 26.1 on p. 312 for a summary of the types of psychiatric admissions)

Voluntary admission
Section 3 of the *MHA*: Here a patient admits himself or herself voluntarily to hospital for treatment. The patient has insight into his or her condition and wants treatment or realizes that he or she needs treatment.

Consent
Section 4 of the *MHA*: Here family members admit a patient, when the patient cannot admit himself or herself, but does not resist admission or treatment.

Reception order (certified admissions)
Section 9 of the *MHA*: Here a patient is admitted to a state mental hospital, and may be kept there for a maximum period of forty-two days. This section is used when patients are mentally ill and lack insight into their condition, and they cannot be treated in the community or in a general hospital, usually because they are either aggressive and violent towards others, or a danger to themselves due to reckless or suicidal behaviour.

A family member or registered health worker (doctor, clinical psychologist, social worker, or professional nurse) fills in the correct form stating why they believe the patient needs admission to a hospital against his or her will. Two qualified medical practitioners must each examine the patient and complete another form. These forms are then submitted to a magistrate (within seven days) who issues a reception order, which then allows the patient to be admitted. This procedure often takes some time, especially in outlying areas, and difficulties may arise with the management of such a patient while waiting for the reception order.

For this reason the law makes provision for an 'urgent admission' under:

Section 12 of the *MHA*: In an emergency, when it is essential that a patient be admitted to a state mental hospital as soon as possible, then a family member or registered health worker (if no family member is available) completes a form and one medical practitioner examines the patient and completes another form. The patient can then be admitted for a maximum of ten days. If it is necessary for them to remain in hospital for a longer period, then the hospital has to arrange for a reception order to be obtained. This involves getting doctors who are not employed there to examine the patient and complete the forms, which is expensive and time-consuming. This section is also the one most likely to be used in an abuse of patient's rights, so all information regarding patients and their behaviour and mental state must be documented as fully as possible, to avoid unpleasant litigation afterwards. Table 26.1 summarizes the various admission procedures.

Table 26.1 Types of psychiatric admissions, detentions, and discharges

Procedure	Process	Conditions/information
1 Voluntary patient (Section 3)		
Admission	• Anyone older than 18 years or the guardian of a patient younger than 18 years can apply.	• Person understands application. • Patient requires treatment.

Table 26.1 continued

Application for discarge	• Medical super-intendent, doctor, or applicant applies for discharge.	• Apply four days before discharge to leave time to obtain reception order should staff not concur.
Discharge	• Discharge by doctor of institution.	

2 Patient by consent (Section 4)

Admission	• Guardian, spouse, near relative, or registered health worker applies. • Report by super-intendent to magistrate.	• Person not opposed to admission but does not under-stand meaning suffi-ciently to be able to apply legally. • Superintendent's report within 7 days of admission. • Magistrate may visit patient.
Application for discharge	• Person who applied for admission.	• Patients may apply personally if they now understand. • Doctor evaluates fit-ness for discharge.
Discharge	• Discharge if fit. • Obtain reception order if dangerous to self or others.	

Table 26.1 continued

3 Reception order (Section 9)

Admission	• Spouse, near relative, or other applies, report by two medical practitioners and magistrate's order.	• Reason to be provided if near relative does not apply. • Nurse may obtain police aid from magistrate if applicable and has problems getting unwilling patient to doctor. • Medical practitioners cannot be partners or relatives. • Certificate not older than 14 days. • Magistrate sees patient, may request witnesses, or additional examination. Apply for reception order within 7 days.
Continued detention	• Reception order with periodical report of medical super-intendent.	• Order valid for 42 days. • Report annually for first 3 years, then in the 5th year, then every 3rd year. • Secretary of Health may investigate.
Discharge	• Doctor discharges or sends out on leave.	• Should patient require readmission while on leave, new certificate not required.

Table 26.1 continued

4 Cases of urgency (Section 12)

Admission	• Near relative older than 18 years or registered health worker; and • One medical practitioner.	• Statement that admission is urgent. • Reasons must be given if someone other than near relative applies. • Certificate not older than 2 days.
Continued detention	• Medical superintendent.	• Admission legal for 10 days only. • Together with additional information (the medical certificate, application for admission)
Discharge	• Magistrate.	• Detention order. • As for Section 9.

Protection afforded by the Act regarding the interests of individuals

Detention of patients

Section 2 of the *MHA* stipulates that mentally ill persons may be detained only in terms of the Act. This provision ensures that all the built-in safety measures of the Act protect such persons from malpractice. Superintendents of licensed institutions are guilty of an offence if they admit or detain more patients than are allowed in terms of the license (Section 61).

Prohibition on sketches, photographs, and false information

Anybody who, without authority, makes or publishes a sketch or photograph of an institution, part of an institution, patient, or group of patients within or outside an institution shall be guilty of an offence. Only the director-general may give written authority for such activity (Section 66 of the *MHA*). This section protects the privacy of psychiatric patients.

Discharge of voluntary patients

Section 5 of the *MHA* provides for the discharge of voluntary patients within four days after the receipt of a written application for discharge. Parents or guardians apply on behalf of patients who are younger than eighteen years. Those who come to hospital voluntarily for treatment may voluntarily leave the hospital.

Patients by consent

The Act protects the interests of patients admitted by consent, in the following ways:

- The doctor who has a patient admitted must be convinced that the patient is not opposed to being admitted.
- The magistrate may visit any patient informally at any time. The magistrate may also investigate the conditions under which patients are admitted or detained and report the findings to the secretary.
- The patient and his or her family should determine the duration of treatment.
- The availability of this type of admission prevents unnecessary certification of patients.

Certification of patients

The certification of patients doesn't depend on the judgment of only one person. The Act makes the following provisions:

- A person who applies for a patient to be certified must be older than eighteen years and preferably a family member. The person must give reasons for the application for a reception order, state his or her relationship to the patient, and verify by affidavit or solemn declaration that the patient had been seen by the person within seven days prior to the date of the application.

- The magistrate must consider the reasons for the application to certify the patient and request examination by two medical practitioners. Their findings must be recorded in the form of a certificate. If the magistrate doubts the degree of mental illness, he or she may summon a witness to testify with regard to the mental condition of the patient. Should the magistrate, upon consideration of all the evidence, find that the patient is not mentally ill, she or he may release him or her.
- Any person who makes false entries or statements in respect of an application for a reception order shall be guilty of an offence.

Issue of certificates by doctors

Section 23 of the *MHA* specifies which medical practitioners may not issue certificates. This measure is aimed at preventing conspiracy and misuse. The following medical practitioners may not issue certificates:

- the applicant for a reception order;
- the family members of a patient;
- the householder of the dwelling to which a patient is to be admitted under a reception order; and
- the guardian or trustee of a patient.

Protection of certified patients

The *curator ad litem* is appointed by the court and acts in the interest of any patient detained in terms of a reception order. The Attorney-General is the official *curator ad litem* of psychiatric patients who are not admitted by consent, within the area for which he or she has been appointed,.

Detainees may apply directly or through the *curator ad litem* to the court for an inquiry into the reasons for their detention. If a person cannot apply personally, a guardian, friend, or family member may apply directly to the court for such an inquiry into the detainee's mental condition (Sections 20 and 21 of the *MHA*).

If the court is convinced that a person who has been detained or declared mentally ill is unable to manage his or her own affairs, it may appoint a *curator bonus* to administer the patient's property. However, if the estimated value of the estate is small, a judge in chambers or the Master of the Supreme Court is appointed to manage the property interests.

Any person who is employed in an institution or other place at which a patient is being detained or who cares for or has charge of a patient and ill-treats or wilfully neglects the patient shall be guilty of an offence (Section 63).

Any person who is employed in an institution or a place of detention and who connives at or incites any person to escape shall be guilty of an offence (Section 64).

A man shall not take personal custody of a female patient or restrain such a patient, except under the continual supervision of a female nurse. This may take place only on the instructions of the superintendent if he or she has reported it to the Director-General. In a case of urgency the superintendent may give his or her consent and report the matter to the Director-General thereafter (Section 65). Any person who has sexual intercourse with a female patient shall be guilty of an offence.

Mechanical means of restraint may not be applied to a patient except where necessary for medical or surgical treatment or to prevent injury to the patient or to others. In both cases a medical certificate describing the mechanical means used and the grounds on which the certificate is founded shall be kept from day to day while it is in use. The notes and the certificate are sent to the Director-General at the end of every quarter (Section 69). Mechanical restraints refer to all instruments and apparatus that restrict or impede the body movements or limbs of a patient. Examples are shackles and strait-jackets. The regulations stipulate that a patient may be kept in isolation only on the prescription of a medical practitioner.

The superintendent or person in charge of the institution in which a patient is detained must send a report of the patient's mental condition to the Director-General annually for the first three years, thereafter the fifth year, and every three years after that. This is done in order to ensure that every patient's condition is thoroughly evaluated at regular intervals. The hospital board visits the institution in which these patients are detained once every two months and offers every patient an opportunity to make representations. The board investigates every reasonable complaint and sends a report of the results of the visit to the Minister. The board also makes recommendations regarding the welfare of these patients.

People who may consent to medical treatment or operations

In terms of the Act certain people may consent to an operation or medical treatment of a mentally ill patient if the patient is incapable of giving consent. The Act provides a priority list of people who may give consent, namely: the curator, the spouse, a parent, a major child, a brother, or a sister. These people will have priority in this order, unless consent is unreasonably withheld or the treatment is urgent and the first person on the list is not available, in which case the next person on the list may give consent.

If none of the listed persons is available, the superintendent of the institution may give written consent if she or he is convinced that the patient's health is at risk (Section 60A).

The superintendent may not consent to sterilization for convenience or to an abortion, unless the health or life of the woman is in danger.

The supervising medical practitioner and relevant therapists may not make unlimited decisions regarding treatment. Regulation 7 was issued in terms of Section 77(1) to regulate the performance of leucotomy on mentally ill patients. There are far more stringent conditions for this procedure than for more usual surgery.

Protection of the community provided by the Act

By means of certain stipulations the Act prevents mentally ill people from becoming a risk or a nuisance to the community.

Duty of medical practitioner regarding notification of dangerous persons

If a medical practitioner examines or treats a person who, in his or her view, is mentally disturbed to such a degree that she or he poses a threat to others, the practitioner must immediately report the matter in writing to the magistrate or a police officer (Section 13).

Certification of psychopaths

A person suffering from a psychopathic disorder may be certified in terms of the Act. The disorder must comply with the definition as set out in the Act:

- It must be a long-term mental disorder.
- It must give rise to irresponsible or abnormal aggression.
- It must have existed before the age of eighteen years.

This protective measure is of great importance, as psychopaths are not certifiable under Section 9.

To prevent dangerous psychopaths from escaping from ordinary psychiatric hospitals, the Act further stipulates that a hospital prison be instituted for psychopaths. This ensures greater safety for the community.

Dangerous patients

Section 27 of the Act states that a state patient or someone in respect of whom a reception order has been issued and who has been found to be dangerous by two medical practitioners, one of whom must be a psychiatrist, shall be referred to a maximum-security hospital or a hospital for psychopaths.

Dangerous behaviour pending certification

Section 12 of the Act provides for an abbreviated reception procedure in cases where there is a risk that a patient may exhibit dangerous behaviour towards himself or herself and others while the reception order is pending.

Application for discharge

The discharge of voluntary patients and patients by consent is preceded by four days' notice. This gives the medical officer time to obtain a reception order if it would be unsafe to discharge the patient.

The Mental Health Act is an improvement on the Mental Disorders Act. Unfortunately the measures aimed at protecting the patient are not always effectively applied. The better nurses know the Act, the more effectively they will be able to apply it to the advantage of individuals and the community.

27 Home visits and record keeping

The primary mental health care nurse, as registered with the South African Nursing Council, is accountable and responsible for her or his acts and/or omissions during nursing care and interactions with the patient. Nurses must record all interactions with their patients, as it is one of the most important requirements of the profession.

Home visits are conducted to assess the patient's mental state and general health, to assess the patient's compliance with medication, and to appraise the patient and his or her family's socio-economic position. The nurse should be able to conduct a home visit and assess the patient, within his or her family, as well as the broader community.

Professional accountability

Professional accountability refers to the responsibility of the nurse (as individual practitioner) for her or his acts and omissions during the nursing care of a patient, or in the performance of any act by the nurse, such as the management of a nursing unit, or education of students. Accountability also implies conditional liability for one's own acts and omissions. The nurse must therefore give account of an act or omission if required to do so. Accountability also implies that the nurse must be willing to be judged according to the rules or professional norms and expectations that have been set and must also bear the consequences of such judgement. Accountability is required on four levels, namely:

- to oneself, i.e. one's own conscience;
- to the patient;
- to the employer; and
- to the courts and the professional council, if necessary.

The patient expects quality nursing and (in terms of the common law principle) expects the nurse to possess all the necessary abilities to perform any nursing interactions. The employer expects quality, cost-effective nursing care, in accordance with the service agreement between employer and employee. As an individual member of the multi-professional health team in the health service, the nurse is personally accountable for her or his acts and omissions.

The individual health practitioner is personally accountable for every act that she or he performs or fails to perform within a multi-professional team context. While there is a shared responsibility for health care, there is also personal or individual liability for the consequences of this care. Every health practitioner has certain functions and responsibilities that are traditionally linked to the specific profession, for example, those of the doctor, pharmacist, nurse, or physiotherapist. However, grey areas also occur in practice, where functions and roles overlap. The available practitioner has an ethical responsibility to act in the interests of the patient, especially if a specific practitioner is absent. This transgression of a practitioner's traditional scope of practice has legal implications and is therefore conditional and regulated by legislation. Therefore, nurses must have personal authorization to prescribe medication to a client or to perform the role of a pharmacist, i.e. to keep and dispense medicine.

Record keeping

The primary professional responsibility for which the nurse can be held liable is the maintenance of the patient's health status. If the nurse does not carry out the prescribed professional responsibilities and this negligence harms a patient, then the professional council may take disciplinary steps against the nurse.

Record keeping is one of the most important requirements that the professional council sets for nurses. Nurses should account in writing for every nurse-patient interaction and should record the results of the interaction. Nurses often neglect this, but it is crucial as all written records are legal documents that can serve as evidence in court cases.

Home visits

Aims

A nurse may need to conduct a home visit for the following reasons:

- to assess the patient's mental state;
- to assess the patient's general health care;
- to assess the patient's compliance with medication;
- to appraise the patient's and family's socio-economic position;
- to appraise the patient's functioning within the family and the influence of interpersonal factors and communication;
- to determine the community resources available to the family;
- to offer support;
- to encourage and motivate the patient and his or her family to participate in the treatment programme;
- to educate the patient, the family, and the public to:
  - understand;
  - accept; and
  - cope with mental illness; or
- to observe cultural patterns and customs and the effect they have on the patient's condition as well as the family's view of mental health and mental illness.

Criteria for home visits

Criteria for home visits to clients include:
- the inability of a patient to attend clinic due to physical illness;
- the nature of a patient's mental state;
- a refusal to attend because the patient:
  - has defaulted; or
  - is psychotic, depressed, etc.
- an emergency, for instance crisis intervention;
- a psychogeriatric assessment (aged, alienated, deluded, depressed, senile patients);
- the administering of medication;
- an appraisal of the home-environment;
- the assistance with or admittance of a patient to hospital;
- the assessment of a patient's functioning within his or her family, i.e. interpersonal factors and communication;
- the assessment of problems and issues that the patient may hide at clinic visits;
- a first visit since discharge;
- an appropriate request by a member of a multidisciplinary team, other organizations, relatives, or members of the community;
- a follow-up visit; or
- a hospital visit.

Home visits concerning certification

- According to the *Mental Health Act* 18 of 1973, the closest family member available *has* to do the certification.
- Any registered or professional health care worker is allowed to do the certification.
- The nurse will only do the certification if there is no family member available, for example if:
  - the family is overseas (not in another province);
  - there are no living relatives; or
  - no other registered professional health care worker is involved with the case.
- The nurse will act as a consultant and will be available for consultation.

Procedure for conducting a home visit

Preparation

If possible the nurse should prepare as follows:

- Confirm that the patient cannot actually come to the clinic himself or herself or send somebody to collect their medication.
- Gather background information.
- Determine a clear reason for the visit.
- Make an appointment, if applicable, to save wasted visits.
- Plan a route.

On arrival

- Identify yourself.
- State the reason for the visit.
- Encourage a relaxed atmosphere to establish rapport.
- Establish a professional relationship (don't take notes during the interview).
- Use yourself as a therapeutic tool: offer kindness, understanding, empathy, and acceptance.
- Use your communication and nursing skills – listen, reflect, etc.
- Avoid overloading the patient; get further information on a later visit.

Observations

Observations should include the patient's:

- background history;
- environment (general cleanliness of patient);
- socio-economic status;
- mental status;
- physical health;
- interpersonal relationships; and
- medication and side effects.

Functioning report

- Schedule follow-up appointments, if appropriate.
- Formulate impressions, views, and opinions for record-keeping.

- Be aware of 'teaching moments', i.e. opportunities to teach the patient and family about the illness, medication, follow-up treatment, and rehabilitation.
- Ensure that visits are goal-orientated.
- Allow time for relationships to develop during first visits.
- Remember you are a guest in the patient's home.
- Don't ever force entry as this can create legal problems.
- If a situation is dangerous (i.e. dogs, firearms, violent patients etc.) do not enter without police assistance.

Record keeping

After the vist, compile an accurate record for the patient's file, including:
- the patient's name;
- your name;
- the date of the visit;
- the time of the visit;
- the patient's problem or need;
- the goal of or reason for the visit;
- your observations;
- the interventions;
- the nursing plan;
- additional information gained from the history form;
- the route form; and
- statistics (e.g. daily follow-ups, males seen, females seen, length of visit)

You should then:
- discuss your findings with members of the multidiscipli-nary team; and
- ensure that you give feedback to the referral source (e.g. the social worker, the occupational therapist, the psychia-trist, or the psychologist).

Appendix 1
ICD–10 Primary Care Version

Categories of mental and behavioural disorders

Code Disorder

Code	Disorder
F00#	Dementia
F05	Delirium
F10	Alcohol use disorders
F11#	Drug use disorders
F17.1	Tobacco use disorders
F20#	Chronic psychotic disorders
F23	Acute psychotic disorders
F31	Bipolar disorder
F32#	Depression
F40	Phobic disorders
F41.0	Panic disorder
F41.1	Generalized anxiety
F41.2	Mixed anxiety and depression
F43.2	Adjustment disorder
F44	Dissociative (conversion) disorder
F45	Unexplained somatic complaints
F48.0	Neurasthenia
F50	Eating disorders
F51	Sleep problems
F52	Sexual disorders
F70	Mental retardation
F90	Hyperkinetic (attention deficit) disorder

Code	Disorder
F91#	Conduct disorder
F98.0	Enuresis
Z63	Bereavement disorders
F99	Mental disorder, not otherwise specified
U50#	Unused/temporarily unassigned to any category

Source: Reprinted from *Diagnostic and Management Guidelines for Mental Disorders in Primary Care: ICD-10 Chapter V Primary Care Version*. Published on behalf of the World Health Organization by Hogrefe & Huber Publishers, 1996.

Appendix 2
DSM-IV – PC Classification Coding Guide

The fourth edition of the *Diagnostic and Statistical Manual of Mental Disorders* (DSM-IV), published by the American Psychiatric Association in 1994 is a multiaxial classification with the following five axes:

AXIS I   Clinical disorders
        Other conditions that may be a focus of clinical attention
AXIS II   Personality disorders
        Mental retardation
AXIS III General medical conditions
AXIS IV Psychosocial and environmental problems
AXIS V   Global assessment of functioning

NOTE: All of the codes provided below are official ICD-9-CM codes. An asterisk (*) after the code indicates that more specific codes to indicate severity and subtypes are available. Refer to the 'Coding and Recording Procedures' sections of the DSM-IV–PC for the specific disorders.

Disorders that commonly present in primary care settings

Depressed mood
293.83	Mood disorder due to a general medical condition
291.8	Alcohol-induced mood disorder
292.84	Other substance-induced (including medication) mood disorder
	Major depressive disorder
296.20*	Single episode
296.30*	Recurrent bipolar I disorder
296.50*	Currently depressed

296.60*	Currently mixed
296.89	Bipolar II disorder
300.4	Dysthymic disorder
v62.82	Bereavement
309.0	Adjustment disorder with depressed mood
309.28	Adjustment disorder with mixed anxiety and depressed mood
311	Depressive disorder not otherwise specified

Anxiety
293.89	Anxiety disorder due to a general medical condition
291.8	Alcohol-induced anxiety disorder
292.89	Other substance-induced (including medication) anxiety disorder
300.21	Panic disorder with agoraphobia
300.01	Panic disorder without agoraphobia
300.23	Social phobia
300.29	Specific phobia
300.22	Agoraphobia without history of panic disorder
309.21	Separation anxiety disorder
300.3	Obsessive-compulsive disorder
309.81	Posttraumatic stress disorder
308.3	Acute stress disorder
300.02	Generalized anxiety disorder
309.24	Adjustment disorder with anxiety
300.00	Anxiety disorder not otherwise specified

Unexplained physical symptoms
300.11	Conversion disorder
300.xx	Pain disorder

307.80	Associated with psychological factors
307.89	Associated with both psychological factors and a general medical condition
300.7	Hypochondriasis
300.7	Body dysmorphic disorder
300.81	Undifferentiated somatoform disorder
300.81	Somatization disorder
v65.2	Malingering
300.19*	Factitious disorder
300.81	Somatoform disorder not otherwise specified

Cognitive disturbance

293.0	Delirium due to a general medical condition
291.0	Alcohol intoxication/ withdrawal delirium
292.81	Other substance intoxication/withdrawal delirium
780.09	Delirium not otherwise specified
	Dementia of the Alzheimer's type
290.10*	With early onset
290.0*	With late onset
290.40*	Vascular dementia
294.1	Dementia due to other general medical conditions
291.2	Alcohol-induced persisting dementia
292.82	Other substance-induced persisting dementia
294.8	Dementia
294.0	Amnestic disorder due to a general medical condition
291.1	Alcohol-induced persisting amnestic disorder
292.83	Other substance-induced persisting amnestic Disorder
294.8	Amnestic disorder not otherwise specified
294.9	Cognitive disorder not otherwise specified

780.9	Age-related cognitive decline
v62.89	Borderline intellectual functioning
319*	Mental retardation, severity unspecified

Problematic substance use

Dependence

303.90	Alcohol dependence
304.40	Amphetamine dependence
304.30	Cannabis dependence
304.20	Cocaine dependence
304.50	Hallucinogen dependence
304.60	Inhalant dependence
305.10	Nicotine dependence
304.00	Opioid dependence
304.90	Phencyclidine dependence
304.10	Sedative, hypnotic, or anxiolytic dependence
304.90	Other (or unknown) dependence

Abuse

305.00	Alcohol abuse
305.70	Amphetamine abuse
305.20	Cannabis abuse
305.60	Cocaine abuse
305.30	Hallucinogen abuse
305.90	Inhalant abuse
305.50	Opioid abuse
305.90	Phencyclidine abuse
305.40	Sedative, hypnotic, or anxiolytic abuse
305.90	Other (or unknown) abuse

Alcohol-induced disorders

303.00	Intoxication
291.8	Withdrawal
291.0	Intoxication/withdrawal delirium
291.2	Persisting dementia
291.1	Persisting amnestic disorder
291.5	Psychotic disorder, with delusions
291.3	Psychotic disorder, with hallucinations
291.8	Mood disorder

291.8	Anxiety disorder
291.8	Sexual dysfunction
291.8	Sleep disorder
291.9	Disorder not otherwise specified

Other substance-induced disorders (other than caffeine)

292.89	Intoxication
292.0	Withdrawal
292.81	Intoxication delirium
292.11	Psychotic disorder, with delusions
292.12	Psychotic disorder, with hallucinations
292.84	Mood disorder
292.89	Anxiety disorder
292.89	Sexual dysfunction
292.89	Sleep disorder
292.9	Other substance-related disorder not otherwise specified

Sleep disturbance

780.59*	Sleep disorder due to a general medical condition
780.59	Breathing-related sleep disorder
291.8	Alcohol-induced sleep disorder
292.89	Other substance-induced (including medication) sleep disorder
307.42	Insomnia related to another mental disorder
307.44	Hypersomnia related to another mental disorder
307.45	Circadian rhythm sleep disorder
307.47	Nightmare disorder
307.46	Sleep Terror disorder
307.46	Sleepwalking disorder
307.47	Parasomnia not otherwise specified
307.42	Primary insomnia
307.44	Primary hypersomnia
307.47	Dyssomnia not otherwise specified

Sexual dysfunction

	Sexual dysfunction due to a general medical condition
625.8*	In a female
608.89*	In a male
291.8	Alcohol-induced sexual dysfunction
292.89	Other substance-induced (including medication) sexual dysfunction
302.71	Hypoactive sexual desire disorder
302.79	Sexual aversion disorder
302.72	Female sexual arousal disorder
302.72	Male erectile disorder
302.73	Female orgasmic disorder
302.74	Male orgasmic disorder
302.75	Premature ejaculation
302.76	Dyspareunia
306.51	Vaginismus
302.70	Sexual dysfunction not otherwise specified

Weight change or abnormal eating

307.1	Anorexia nervosa
307.51	Bulimia nervosa
307.50	Eating disorder not otherwise specified

Psychotic symptoms

293.81	Psychotic disorder due to a general medical condition, with delusions
293.82	Psychotic disorder due to a general medical condition, with hallucinations
293.0	Delirium due to a general medical condition
	Dementia of the Alzheimer's Type
290.10*	With early onset
290.0*	With late onset
290.40*	Vascular dementia
294.1	Dementia due to a general medical condition

291.0	Alcohol intoxication delirium
291.0	Alcohol withdrawal delirium
292.81	Other substance intoxication delirium
292.81	Sedative/other substance withdrawal delirium
291.2	Alcohol-induced persisting dementia
292.82	Inhalant/other substance-induced persisting dementia
296.44	Bipolar I disorder, most recent episode manic, severe with psychotic features
296.54	Bipolar I disorder, most recent episode depressed, severe with psychotic features
296.24	Major depressive disorder, single episode, severe with psychotic features
296.34	Major depressive disorder, recurrent, severe with psychotic features
298.8	Brief psychotic disorder
295.90*	Schizophrenia
295.40	Schizophreniform disorder
295.70	Schizoaffective disorder
297.1	Delusional disorder
298.9	Psychotic disorder not otherwise specified

Psychosocial problems

Psychological and behavioral factors that affect health care

| 316 | Psychological factors affecting a medical condition |
| v15.81 | Noncompliance with treatment |

Relational (family) problems

| v61.9 | Relational problem related to a mental disorder or a medical condition |

v61.20	Parent-child relational problem
v61.1	Partner relational problem
v61.8	Sibling relational problem
v61.81	Relational problem not otherwise specified

Problems related to abuse or neglect

v61.21	Physical abuse of child
v61.21	Sexual abuse of child
v61.21	Neglect of child
v61.1	Physical abuse of adult
v61.1	Sexual abuse of adult

Problems related to personal roles

v62.89	Phase of life problem
313.82	Identity problem
v62.89	Religious or spiritual problem
v62.2	Occupational problem

Social problems

v60.9	Housing problem
v60.9	Economic problem
v63.9	Problems with access to health care services
v62.5	Problems related to interaction with the legal system/crime
v62.4	Acculturation problem

Problems listed in other sections

v62.82	Bereavement
v62.89	Borderline intellectual functioning
v62.3	Academic problem
v71.02	Child or adolescent antisocial behavior
v71.01	Adult antisocial behavior
v65.2	Malingering
780.9	Age-related cognitive decline

Other mental disorders

Manic symptoms

| 293.83 | Mood disorder due to a general medical condition |

291.8	Alcohol-induced mood disorder
292.84	Other substance-induced (including medication) mood disorder
	Bipolar I disorder
296.00*	Single manic episode
296.40*	Recurrent, currently manic
296.60*	Recurrent, currently mixed
296.7	Most recent episode unspecified
296.89	Bipolar II disorder
301.13	Cyclothymic disorder
296.80	Bipolar disorder not otherwise specified

Impulse-control symptoms

312.34	Intermittent explosive disorder
312.32	Kleptomania
312.33	Pyromania
312.31	Pathological gambling
312.39	Trichotillomania
312.30	Impulse-control disorder not otherwise specified

Deviant sexual arousal

302.81	Fetishism
302.3	Transvestic fetishism
302.4	Exhibitionism
302.82	Voyeurism
302.2	Pedophilia
302.83	Sexual masochism
302.84	Sexual sadism
302.89	Frotteurism
302.9	Paraphilia not otherwise specified

Dissociative symptoms

300.12	Dissociative amnesia
300.13	Dissociative fugue
300.14	Dissociative identity disorder
300.6	Depersonalization disorder
300.15	Dissociative disorder dot otherwise specified

Abnormal movements/ vocalizations

307.23	Tourette's disorder
307.22	Chronic motor or vocal tic disorder
307.21	Transient tic disorder
307.20	Tic disorder not otherwise specified
307.3	Stereotypic movement disorder
293.89	Catatonic disorder due to a general medical condition

Dysfunctional personality traits

Cluster A:

301.0	Paranoid personality disorder
301.20	Schizoid personality disorder
301.22	Schizotypal personality disorder

Cluster B:

301.7	Antisocial personality disorder
301.83	Borderline personality disorder
301.50	Histrionic personality disorder
301.81	Narcissistic personality disorder

Cluster C:

301.82	Avoidant personality disorder
301.6	Dependent personality disorder
301.4	Obsessive-compulsive personality disorder

Other disorders related to personality:

301.9	Personality disorder not otherwise specified
310.1	Personality change due to a general medical condition

Disorders usually first diagnosed in infancy, childhood, or adolescence

Intellectual functioning disorders

317	Mild mental retardation
318.0	Moderate mental retardation
318.1	Severe mental retardation
318.2	Profound mental retardation
319	Mental retardation, severity unspecified
v62.89	Borderline intellectual functioning

Academic skills disorders

315.00	Reading disorder
315.1	Mathematics disorder
315.2	Disorder of written expression
315.9	Learning disorder not otherwise specified
v62.3	Academic problem

Motor skills disorder

315.4	Developmental coordination disorder

Disruptive behavior and inattention

314.xx	Attention-deficit/hyperactivity disorder
314.01	Combined type
314.00	Predominantly-inattentive type
314.01	Predominantly hyperactive-impulsive type
314.9	Attention-deficit/hyperactivity disorder not otherwise specified

Negative/antisocial behavior

312.8*	Conduct disorder
313.81	Oppositional defiant disorder
312.9	Disruptive behavior
	disorder not otherwise specified
v71.02	Child or adolescent antisocial behavior

Feeding, eating, or elimination

307.6	Enuresis
– · –	Encopresis
787.6	With constipation and overflow incontinence
307.7	Without constipation and overflow incontinence
307.52	Pica
307.53	Rumination disorder
307.59	Feeding disorder of infancy or early childhood

Communication disorders

315.31	Expressive language disorder
315.31	Mixed receptive-expressive language disorder
315.39	Phonological disorder
307.0	Stuttering
307.9	Communication disorder not otherwise specified

Impaired social interaction

299.00	Autistic disorder
299.80	Rett's disorder
299.10	Childhood distintegrative disorder
299.80	Asperger's disorder
299.80	Pervasive development disorder not otherwise specified
313.23	Selective mutism
313.89	Reactive attachment disorder of infancy or early childhood

Gender identity disorders

302.6	Gender identity disorder in children
302.85	Gender identity disorder in adolescents or adults

SOURCE: Reprinted from the
Diagnostic and Statistical Manual of
Mental Disorders – Primary care
version, fourth edition. Copyright
1994 American Psychiatric
Association

Glossary

Aa

acute intoxication a transient condition, following the administration of a psychoactive substance, causing changes in physiological, psychological, or behavioural functions and responses.

affect pattern of observable behaviours, which is the expression of a subjectively experienced feeling state (emotion), and is variable over time, in response to changing emotional states.

agitation excessive motor activity with a feeling of inner tension.

agnosic alexia words can be seen but not read.

agoraphobia literally a fear of the market place. A generalized high anxiety level with multiple phobic symptoms occurs. It may include a fear of crowds, open and closed spaces, and travelling by public transport.

alexithymia difficulty in being aware of, or describing, one's emotions.

ambivalence simultaneous presence of opposing impulses towards the same thing.

amnesia inability to recall past experiences.

amok seen in south-east Asia. There is an outburst of aggressive behaviour, in which the patient runs amok, following a depressive episode.

anhedonia inability to feel enjoyment.

anosognosia lack of awareness of disease.

anxiety feeling of apprehension or tension caused by anticipating an external or internal danger.

apathy detachment or indifference, and a loss of emotional tone and the ability to feel pleasure.

attention ability to focus on an activity.

automatism act over which a person has no control, e.g. sleepwalking.

Bb

blunted affect reduction in emotional expression.

Cc

Capgras' syndrome a person who is familiar to the patient is believed to have been replaced by a double.

central (syntactical) aphasia difficulty in arranging words in their correct sequence.

circumstantiality slowed thinking incorporating unnecessary trivial details. The goal of thought is finally, but slowly, reached.

clanging speech in which words are chosen because of their sounds rather than their meanings. It includes rhyming and punning.

clouding of consciousness the patient is drowsy and does not react completely to stimuli. There is disturbance of attention, concentration, memory, orientation and thinking.

coma in deep coma there is no response to deep pain or any spontaneous movement. Tendon, pupillary, and corneal reflexes are usually absent.

compulsions or compulsive rituals repetitive, stereotyped, seemingly purposeful behaviour that is the motor component of obsessive thoughts, e.g. checking and cleaning rituals.

concentration ability to sustain attention.

concrete thinking lack of abstract thinking, normal in childhood, and occurring in adults with organic brain disease and schizophrenia.

confabulation gaps in memory are unconsciously filled with false memories.

Cotard's syndrome nihilistic delusional disorder in which, for example, patients believe their money, friends, or body parts do not exist.

countertransference therapist's emotions and attitudes to the patient.

culture-bound syndromes specific psychiatric disorders occurring in certain non-Western countries.

Dd

defence mechanisms mental mechanisms that protect consciousness from the affects, ideas, and desires of the unconscious.

déjà pensé illusion of recognition of a situation.

déjà vu illusion of recognition of a new thought.

delirium disorder of consciousness in which the patient is bewildered, disoriented, and restless. There may be associated fear and hallucinations.

delusions of infidelity (pathological jealousy, delusional jealousy, Othello's syndrome) delusional belief that one's spouse or lover is being unfaithful.

delusion of reference behaviour of others, and objects and events, e.g. television broadcasts, believed to refer to oneself in particular. When similar thoughts are held with less than delusional intensity they are ideas of reference.

delusion false personal belief based on incorrect inference about external reality and firmly sustained in spite of both what almost everyone else believes and what constitutes incontrovertible and obvious proof or evidence to the contrary. The belief is not one normally held by others of the same subculture.

delusional perception new and delusional significance is attached to a familiar real perception without any logical reason.

dementia global organic impairment of intellectual functioning without impairment of consciousness.

denial defence mechanism in which the subject acts as if consciously unaware of a wish or reality.

dependence syndrome use of psychoactive substances has a higher priority than other behaviours that once had higher value. There is a desire, often strong and overpowering, to take the substance(s) on a continuous or periodic basis.

depersonalization feeling that one is altered or not real in some way.

depression low or depressed mood that may be accompanied by anhedonia, in which the ability to enjoy regular and pleasurable activities is lost. In normal grief or mourning, the sadness is appropriate to the loss.

derealization surroundings do not seem real.

disorders (loosening) of association (formal thought disorder) language disorder seen in schizophrenia, e.g. knight's move thinking and word salad.

dissociative disorder disorder in which there is a disturbance in the normal integration of awareness of identity, consciousness, memory and control of bodily movements.

distractibility attention is frequently drawn to irrelevant external stimuli.

DSM-IV fourth edition of the *Diagnostic and Statistical Manual of Mental Disorders*, published by the American Psychiatric Association, Washington DC (1994). It is a multiaxial classification with 5 axes.

dysarthria difficulty articulating speech.

dysphoria unpleasant mood.

Ee

echolalia automatic imitation of another's speech.

echopraxia automatic imitation of another's movements occurring even when asked not to.

ecstasy feeling of intense rapture.

ego part of the mental apparatus that is present at the interface of the perceptual and internal demand systems. It controls voluntary thoughts and actions and, at an unconscious level, defence mechanisms.

eidetic image vivid and detailed reproduction of a previous perception, e.g. a photographic memory.

elevated mood mood more cheerful than normal. It is not necessarily pathological.

erotomania (de Clérambault's syndrome) patient holds the delusional belief that someone else, usually of a higher social or professional status, is in love with them.

euphoric mood exaggerated feeling of well-being. It is pathological.

expansive mood feelings are expressed without restraint, and one's self-importance may be overrated.

expressive (motor) aphasia difficulty in expressing thoughts in words while comprehension remains.

extracampine hallucination hallucination occurring outside one's sensory field.

Ff

fear anxiety caused by a recognized real danger.

flat affect almost no emotional expression at all; the patient typically has an immobile face and monotonous voice.

flight of ideas speech consists of a stream of accelerated thoughts with abrupt changes from topic to topic and no central direction. The connections between the thoughts may be based on chance relationships, verbal associations (e.g. alliteration and assonance), clang associations, and distracting stimuli.

formication somatic hallucination in which insects are felt to be crawling under one's skin.

free association articulation, without censorship, of all thoughts that come to mind.

free-floating anxiety pervasive and unfocused anxiety.

Fregoli's syndrome patient believes that a familiar person, who is often believed to be the patient's persecutor, has taken on different appearances.

fugue state of wandering from usual surroundings and loss of memory.

functional hallucination stimulus causing the hallucination is experienced in addition to the hallucination.

Gg

global aphasia both receptive and expressive aphasia present at the same time.

Hh

hallucination false sensory perception in the absence of a real external stimulus. It is perceived as being located in objective space and as having the same realistic qualities as normal perceptions. It is not subject to conscious manipulation and only indicates a psychotic disturbance when there is also impaired reality testing.

hallucinosis hallucinations (usually auditory) occurring in clear conscious, e.g. in alcoholism.

hemisomatognosis (hemidepersonalization) limb is felt to be missing.

hyperacusis increased sensitivity to sounds.

hyperaesthesia sensory distortion in which sensations appear increased.

hyperkinesis overactivity, distractibility, excitability, and impulsivity, e.g. in children.

hypnogogic hallucination hallucination occurring while falling asleep. It occurs in normal people.

hypnopompic hallucination hallucination occurring while waking from sleep. It occurs in normal people.

hypoaesthesia sensory distortion in which sensations appear decreased.

hypochondriasis preoccupation, not based on real organic pathology, with a fear of having a serious physical illness. Physical sensations are unrealistically interpreted as being abnormal.

Ii

ICD-10 tenth revision of the *International Classification of Diseases* published by the World Health Organization, Geneva (1992).

ideas of reference see under *delusion of reference*.

illusion false perception of a real external stimulus.

inappropriate affect affect that is inappropriate to the
. circumstances, for example, appearing cheerful immediately following the death of a loved one.

induced psychosis (folie à deux) delusional disorder shared by two (or more) people who are closely related emotionally. One has a genuine psychotic disorder and his or her delusional system is induced in the other, who may be dependent or less intelligent.

Jj

jamais vu illusion of failure to recognize a familiar situation.

jargon aphasia incoherent, meaningless, neologistic speech occurs.

Kk

Kluver-Bucy syndrome syndrome characterized by placidity, hyper-orality, hypersexuality, hyper-metamorphosis, and hyperphagia, resulting from bilateral destruction of the amygdaloid bodies of the limbic system.

knight's move thinking odd, tangential associations between ideas leading to disruptions in the smooth continuity of speech.

Ll

labile affect affect repeatedly and rapidly shifts, for example, from sadness to anger.

learning disability (mental retardation) classified by DSM-IV and ICD-10 as an intelligence quotient of 70 or less.

logoclonia last syllable of the last word is repeated.

logorrhoea (volubility) fluent and rambling speech using many words.

Mm

macropsia objects appear larger or nearer.

mannerisms repeated, involuntary movements that appear to be goal directed.

mens rea guilty state of mind at the time of a criminal offence.

micropsia objects appear smaller or farther away.

mild mental retardation intelligence quotient of 50–70 (inclusive).

moderate mental retardation intelligence quotient of 35-49 (inclusive).

monomania pathological preoccupation with a single object.

mood pervasive and sustained emotion, which, in the extreme, markedly colours the person's perception of the world.

mood congruent delusion content of the delusion is appropriate to the patient's mood.

mood incongruent delusion content of the delusion is inappropriate to the patient's mood.

mutism total loss of speech.

Nn

negativism motiveless resistance to commands and attempts to be moved.

neologism word newly made up, or an everyday word used in a special way.

neurosis neurotic disorder that is a psychiatric disorder in which the patient has insight into the illness, has only part of his or her personality involved in the disorder, can distinguish between subjective experiences and reality, and does not construct a false environment based on misconceptions.

nihilistic delusion delusion belief that others, oneself or the world does not exist or is about to cease to exist.

nominal aphasia difficulty in naming objects.

Oo

obsessions repetitive, senseless thoughts recognized as being irrational by the patient, which, at least initially, are unsuccessfully resisted.

overvalued idea unreasonable and sustained intense preoccupation maintained with less than delusional intensity. The belief is demonstrably false and not one normally held by others of the same subculture. There is a marked associated emotional investment.

Pp

palilalia word is repeated with increasing frequency.

panic attacks acute, episodic, intense anxiety attacks with or without physiological symptoms.

pareidolia vivid imagery occurring without conscious effort while looking at a poorly-structured background.

paramnesia distorted recall leading to falsification of memory, e.g. confabulation, *déjà vu, déjà pensé, jamais vu,* retrospective falsification.

passing by the point (vorbeigehen) answers to questions, though obviously wrong, show that the questions have been understood, e.g. asked 'What colour is grass?', the patient may answer 'Blue'. It is seen in Ganser's syndrome, first described in criminals awaiting trial.

passivity phenomena delusional belief that an external agency is controlling aspects of the self that are normally entirely under one's own control (e.g. thought alienation, made feelings, made impulses, made actions, somatic passivity).

perseveration (of speech and movement) mental operations carry on beyond the point at which they are appropriate.

personality disorders deeply ingrained and enduring behaviour patterns manifesting as inflexible responses to a broad range of personal and social situations.

phantom limb following the removal of a limb there is a continued awareness of its presence.

phobia persistent irrational fear of an activity, object, or situation leading to avoidance. The fear is out of proportion to the real danger and cannot be reasoned away, being out of voluntary control.

phobic anxiety focus of anxiety is avoided.

physical dependence adaptive state in which intense physical disturbance occurs when the administration of a psychoactive substance is suspended. There is a desire to take the substance to avoid the physical symptoms of the withdrawal state.

posturing an inappropriate or bizarre bodily posture adopted continuously over a long period.

poverty of speech very reduced speech sometimes with mono-syllabic answers to questions.

pressure of speech increased quantity and rate of speech that is difficult to interrupt.

primary delusion delusion arising fully formed without any discernible connection with previous events. It may be preceded by a delusional mood in which there is an awareness of something unusual and threatening occurring.

profound mental retardation intelligence quotient of less than 20.

prosopagnosia inability to recognize faces.

pseudodementia similar clinically to dementia but has a non-organic cause, e.g. depression.

pseudohallucination form of imagery arising in the subjective inner space of the mind and lacking the substantiality of normal perceptions. It is not subject to conscious manipulation.

psychological dependence psycho-active substance producing a feeling of satisfaction and a psychological drive that requires periodic or continuous administration of the substance to produce pleasure, or to avoid the psychological discomfort of its absence.

psychomotor agitation excess (usually unproductive) over-activity and restlessness, e.g. in agitated depression.

psychosis psychotic disorder in which the patient does not have insight, has the whole of his or her personality distorted by illness, and constructs a false environment out of subjective experiences. Delusions and/or hallucinations may occur.

pure word deafness words that are heard cannot be comprehended.

Rr

rationalization defence mechanism in which an attempt is made to explain in a logically consistent or ethically acceptable way affects, ideas, and wishes the true motive of which is not consciously perceived.

receptive (sensory) aphasia difficulty in comprehending word meanings.

reduplication phenomenon part or all the body is felt to be duplicated.

reflex hallucination stimulus in one sensory field leads to a hallucination in another sensory field.

regression defence mechanism in which there is a return to an earlier stage of development.

repression defence mechanism in which there is a pushing away of unacceptable affects, ideas, and wishes so that they remain in the unconscious.

retrospective falsification false details are added to the recollection of an otherwise real memory.

Ss

selective inattention anxiety-provoking stimuli are blocked out.

semi-coma semi-comatose patient withdraws the source of pain but does not show spontaneous motor activity.

severe mental retardation intelligence quotient of 20–34 (inclusive).

simple phobia fear of discrete objects (e.g. spiders) or situations.

social phobia fear of personal interactions in a public setting, e.g. public speaking and eating in public.

somnambulism sleep walking.

somnolence patient who is drowsy or somnolent can be awoken by mild stimuli and can speak comprehensibly, perhaps for

only a short while before falling asleep again.

stammering flow of speech is broken by pauses and the repetition of parts of words.

stereotype repeated, regular fixed pattern of movement or speech that is not goal directed.

synaesthesia stimulus in one sensory field leading to hallucination in another sensory field.

systematized delusion group of delusions united by a single theme or a delusion with multiple elaborations.

Tt

tactile (haptic) hallucinations superficial somatic hallucinations.

talking past the point (vorbeireden) point of what is being said is never quite reached.

tangential thoughts rambling thoughts leading off the subject never coming to the point.

tension unpleasant increase in psychomotor activity.

thought alienation delusional belief that one's thoughts are under the control of an outside agency or that others are participating in one's thinking. It includes thought insertion, thought withdrawal, and thought broadcasting.

thought blocking sudden interruption in the train of thought, leaving a 'blank', after which what was being said cannot be recalled.

thought broadcasting delusional belief that one's thoughts are being 'read' by others, as if they were being broadcast.

thought insertion delusional belief that thoughts are being put into one's mind by an external agency.

thought withdrawal delusional belief that thoughts are being removed from one's mind by an external agency.

tics repeated, irregular movements involving a muscle group.

tolerance desired central nervous system effects of a psychoactive substance diminish with repeated use, so that increasing doses are needed to achieve the same effects.

trailing phenomenon moving objects are seen as a series of discrete discontinuous images. It is associated with hallucinations.

Vv

visceral hallucinations somatic hallucinations of deep sensations.

visual asymbolia words can be transcribed but not read.

Ww

wavy flexibility (cerea flexibilitas) the examiner, as he or she moves part of the patient's body, has a feeling of plastic resistance as if bending of a soft wax rod. The bodily part remains 'moulded' in its new position.

withdrawal state physical and psychological symptoms, which may be complicated by delirium or convulsions, occur following absolute or relative withdrawal of a psychoactive substance after its repeated use.

word salad (schizophasia or speech confusion) the speech is an incoherent and incomprehensible mix of words and phrases.

Source: Reprinted from *Saunders' pocket essentials of psychiatry* by Basant K. Puri, 1995, by permission of the author and the publisher WB Saunders Company Limited.

Select bibliography

Allwood, G.W. & Gagiano, C.A. 1997. *Handbook of psychiatry for primary care.* Cape Town: Oxford University Press.

American Association on Mental Retardation. 1992. *The ad hoc committee on terminology and classification.* Washington, DC: The Association.

American Psychiatric Association. 1994. *Diagnostic and statistical manual of mental disorders.* 4th ed. Washington, DC: American Psychiatric Press.

American Psychiatric Association. 1994. *Diagnostic and statistical manual of mental disorders*: primary care version. (4th edn.) Washington, DC: American Psychiatric Press.

Andreasen, N.C. & Black, D.W. 1995. *Introductory textbook of psychiatry.* (2nd edn.) Washington, DC: American Psychiatric Press.

Anthony, W., Cohen, M. & Farkas, M. 1990. *Psychiatric rehabilitation.* Boston: Boston University Press.

Clews, F. & Thom, R. 1999. *Primary mental health care, a trainer's manual.* Centre for Health Policy: University of Witwatersrand.

Coffey, C.E. & Cummings, J.L. 1994. *Textbook of geriatric neuropsychiatry.* Washington, DC: American Psychiatric Press.

Dinkmeyer, D., McKay, G.P. & Dinkmeyer, J.S. 1997. *The parents handbook – systematic training for effective parenting.* American Guidance Service.

Di Vasto, P.V., Weat, D.A. & Christy, J.G. 1979. A framework for the emergency evaluation of the suicidal patient. In *Journal of psychiatric nursing and mental health services.* June: 15–20.

Engel, G.L. 1980. The clinical application of the biopsychosocial model. *American Journal of Psychiatry* 137: 535–544.

Evian, C. 1993. *Primary Aids care – a practical guide for primary health care personnel.* Johannesburg: Jacana.

Gelder, M. *et al.* 1994. *Oxford textbook of psychiatry.* (2nd. edn.) Oxford: Oxford University Press.

Gmeiner, A.C. 1998. *Facilitating communication – how to improve communication skillls to achieve successful results.* Continuing center for education. California.

Kaplan, H.I. *et al.* 1994. Clinical examination of the psychiatric patient. In *Synopsis of psychiatry* ed. by H.I. Kaplan *et al.* (7th edn.) Baltimore: Williams & Wilkins: 267–299.

Madela, E. 2000. 'Scope of mental health at primary mental health care level', unpublished.

Madela-Mntla, E.N., Poggenpoel, M. and Gmeiner, A.C. 1999. 'A model for culture – congruent psychiatric nursing' in *Curationis*, September 1999.

Kaplan, H.I.1994. The doctor-patient relationship and interviewing techniques. In *Synopsis of psychiatry* ed. by H.I.

Kaplan *et al.* (7th edn.) Baltimore: Williams & Wilkins 1–15.

Kaplan, H.I. & Sadock, B.J. 1996. *Synopsis of psychiatry.* (8th edn.) Williams & Wilkins.

Mbiti, J.S. 1991. *Introduction to African Religions.* (2nd edn.) New Hampshire: Heineman

Meiring, P. de V. 1990. *Textbook of geriatric medicine.* Cape Town: Juta.

Pitt, B. 1974. *Psychogeriatrics: an introduction to the psychiatry of old age.* Edinburgh: Livingstone.

Perko, J.E. & Kreigh, H.Z. 1988. *Psychiatric and mental health nursing – a commitment to care and concern.* New Jersey: Prentice-Hall.

Puri, B.K. 1995. *Saunders' pocket essentials of psychiatry.* London: W.B. Saunders.

Rawlins, R.P. & Heacok, P.E. 1993. *Clinical manual of psychiatric nursing.* Mosby.

Strauss, G.D. 1995. Diagnosis and psychiatry: examination of the psychiatric patient. In *comprehensive textbook of psychiatry* ed. by H.I. Kaplan *et al.* (6th edn). Baltimore: Williams & Wilkins.

Tomb, D.A. 1995. *Psychiatry.* (5th edn.) Baltimore: Williams & Wilkins.

Uys, L. & Middleton, L. (eds.). 1997. *Mental health nursing – a South African perspective.* Juta.

Uys, L.R. 1995. *Primary psychiatric care course 2: Rehabilitation.* University of Natal: Unpublished manual.

van Luyn, J.B. *et al.* 1992. *Emergency psychiatry today.* Amsterdam: Elsevier.

Wilkinson, J.N. 1991. *Nursing process in action – a critical thinking approach.* Addison-Wesley.

Wilson, H.S. & Kneisl, C.R. 1996. *Psychiatric nursing.* (5th edn.) California: Addison-Wesley.

Index